Animal Restraint for Veterinary Professionals

Animal Restraint for Veterinary Professionals

Second Edition

C.C. Sheldon, DVM, MS
Instructor, Veterinary Technician Program
Madison Area Technical College
Madison, Wisconsin

Teresa F. Sonsthagen, BS, LVT
Instructor, Veterinary Technology Program
North Dakota State University
Fargo, North Dakota

James A. Topel, CVT
Instructor, Veterinary Technician Program
Madison Area Technical College
Madison, Wisconsin

With 547 color illustrations

ELSEVIER

ELSEVIER

3251 Riverport Lane
Maryland Heights, Missouri 63043

ANIMAL RESTRAINT FOR VETERINARY PROFESSIONALS,
SECOND EDITION   ISBN: 978-0-323-35494-3

Notices

Knowledge and best practice in this field are constantly changing. As new research and experience broaden
our understanding, changes in research methods, professional practices, or medical treatment may become
necessary.

Practitioners and researchers must always rely on their own experience and knowledge in evaluating and
using any information, methods, compounds, or experiments described herein. In using such information
or methods they should be mindful of their own safety and the safety of others, including parties for whom
they have a professional responsibility.

With respect to any drug or pharmaceutical products identified, readers are advised to check the most
current information provided (i) on procedures featured or (ii) by the manufacturer of each product to be
administered, to verify the recommended dose or formula, the method and duration of administration, and
contraindications. It is the responsibility of practitioners, relying on their own experience and knowledge of
their patients, to make diagnoses, to determine dosages and the best treatment for each individual patient,
and to take all appropriate safety precautions.

To the fullest extent of the law, neither the Publisher nor the authors, contributors, or editors assume any
liability for any injury and/or damage to persons or property as a matter of products liability, negligence or
otherwise, or from any use or operation of any methods, products, instructions, or ideas contained in the
material herein.

Library of Congress Cataloging-in-Publication Data

Names: Sheldon, C.C. | Sonsthagen, Teresa F. | Topel, James.
Title: Animal restraint for veterinary professionals/C.C. Sheldon, DVM, MS,
   instructor, Veterinary Technician Program, Madison Area Technical College,
   Madison, Wisconsin, Teresa F. Sonsthagen, BS, LVT, instructor, Veterinary
   Technology Program, North Dakota State University, Fargo, North Dakota,
   James A. Topel, CVT, instructor, Veterinary Technician Program, Madison
   Area Technical College, Madison, Wisconsin.
Description: Second edition. | Maryland Heights, Missouri : Elsevier, [2017]
   | "With 547 color illustrations." | Includes index.
Identifiers: LCCN 2016019314 | ISBN 9780323354943 (pbk.)
Subjects: LCSH: Animal immobilization.
Classification: LCC SF760.A55 S54 2017 | DDC 636.089–dc23 LC record available at
   https://lccn.loc.gov/2016019314

Content Strategist: Brandi Graham
Content Development Manager: Luke Held
Content Development Specialist: Jennifer Bertucci
Publishing Services Manager: Hemamalini Rajendrababu
Project Manager: Andrea Lynn Villamero
Designer: Margaret Reid

Printed in China
Last digit is the print number: 9 8 7 6 5 4 3 2 1

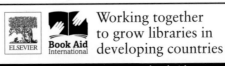

For those who have lost their temper, their skin, or their cool while restraining an animal and for students, past, present, and future—may you always hear these words: "Who has control of that dog's head?"

To the animals of the world, we owe our gratitude. You make our lives so much richer. May we treat you all with respect and compassion.

This book was designed to provide a pictorial guide to common animal restraints. This text demonstrates accepted veterinary handling and restraint techniques drawn from our personal experiences and time-tested handling and restraint techniques used by the veterinary profession. It also integrates handling and restraint theory with step-by-step discussion and digital camera images. We hope that this text can be used both as a resource for veterinary students and veterinary technician students and as a reference for the "experienced" veterinary professional. In our experience, understanding animal behavior is paramount when refining animal restraint techniques. We hope that this text is used in conjunction with the many references available on animal behavior.

The text has been divided into an introduction, a chapter on knots used for restraint, and nine chapters discussing handling and restraint techniques for the more common animals seen in the veterinary clinic and visited on farm calls. In addition, resources are included at the end of each chapter that may be referenced for additional handling and restraint techniques used in the veterinary profession.

We acknowledge that every animal is unique and each restraint situation must be handled differently. Both animal and handler stress can be reduced through calm preparation and better understanding of animal behavior. Though individual restraint techniques may vary among veterinary practitioners, the common theme of safety for human and animal must underlie all restraint. Inherent to all animal restraint is the understanding of animal behavior so that we can continually refine our technique to improve the animal's and handler's experience. A lifelong study of animal behavior is required for all who work with animals.

One of the authors' neighbors is a volunteer firefighter. Every Thursday for over 30 years he has gone to the firehouse to practice hooking up fire hoses to the fire truck. We believe he knows how to hook a fire hose to the truck. We also believe that through repetition mechanical tasks can become second nature in an emergency situation. This is true of animal restraint as well. Practice in the calm times so that in times of stress or in emergency situations your actions demonstrate proficiency.

Practice makes perfect.

C.C. Sheldon
Teresa F. Sonsthagen
James A. Topel

ACKNOWLEDGMENTS

To those animals whose pictures appear in this book, THANK YOU!!! You are the best teachers ever.

A very special thank you to the associates at Brodhead Veterinary Medical Center in Brodhead, WI; Spring Grove Dairy in Brodhead, WI; and Melissa Clarke for providing photographs.

CONTENTS

1   Restraint Principles, 1

2   Knot Tying, 7

3   Restraint of Cats, 23

4   Restraint of Dogs, 55

5   Restraint of Cattle, 107

6   Restraint of Horses, 131

7   Restraint of Sheep, 159

8   Restraint of Goats, 169

9   Restraint of Swine, 177

10 Restraint of Rodents, Rabbits, and Ferrets, 187

11 Restraint of Birds, 219

APPENDIX A Gender Names, 229

APPENDIX B Physiologic Data, 231

Glossary, 233

Index, 235

1

Restraint Principles

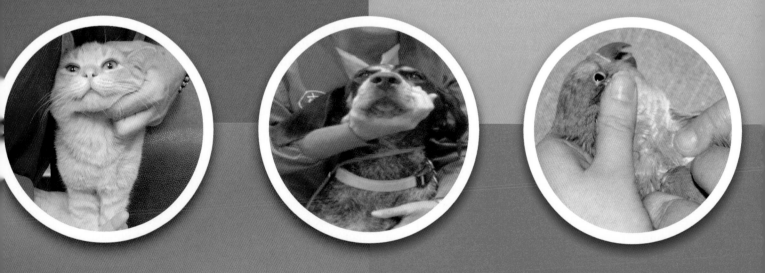

WHY LEARN RESTRAINT TECHNIQUES?

Veterinary medicine is dedicated to the preservation of the health and well-being of animals. As in human medicine, this involves a variety of diagnostic and therapeutic procedures. But unlike human patients, veterinary patients are not willing to have blood samples drawn or to hold perfectly still for radiographs, and sometimes even resent being touched! Therefore, as veterinary professionals, we must learn how to properly restrain our patients.

Restraint means the holding back, checking, or suppressing of action; keeping under control; or depriving of physical freedom. Various degrees of patient restraint can be used to allow the veterinary medical team to examine, treat, and perform supportive procedures on the patient as prescribed by the veterinarian. Restraint in its mildest form is a gentle touch and a soft voice. For example, when first meeting a canine patient, you need to start with a soft stroke to the head and a gentle hello. This will go a long way in gaining that animal's trust.

In its moderate form, restraint can involve confinement in a corral, box stall, or cage that limits the animal's movement or may be as restrictive as immobilizing a portion of the animal's body, as is necessary for jugular venipuncture. Restraint in its most restrictive form can be as involved as causing a reduction or complete loss of muscular control through use of chemicals such as tranquilizers, sedatives, and general anesthetics.

CONSIDERATIONS FOR RESTRAINT

Some basic guidelines should be kept in mind while you are learning and performing restraint techniques on animals: How will the restraint technique affect the animal? Is the selected restraint technique safe for the people and animal involved? What technique and equipment should be used? When and where should the restraint procedure be done? Who should perform the restraint procedure?

EFFECTS OF RESTRAINT ON ANIMALS

The goal in any restraint procedure is to minimize the effects of handling. Improper restraint can affect an animal physically and/or psychologically for the rest of its life. For this reason, it is our responsibility to contain our temper, use good judgment in matching the restraint technique with the individual, and apply the minimum amount of restraint necessary to complete the procedure.

SAFETY CONSIDERATIONS

Human Safety

It is important to ensure the safety of the people involved in any restraint procedure, not only to maintain their health, but also for economic reasons. Injury to veterinary personnel means loss of income for the practice, and injury to an animal owner can result in a lawsuit. Before you apply any restraint to an animal, you must ask yourself two important questions if you are to prevent injury.

Question 1: What type of animal behavior am I dealing with?

Knowing animals' normal behavior patterns provides you with important information on what can make them nervous or frightened and enables you to predict how they are likely to react in a particular situation.

All animals, including humans, operate under the "fight-or-flight" principle. The basic premise is, "If I feel threatened and can't get away from my attacker, then I will fight to preserve my life." In predator species such as dogs and cats, we must keep the animal from thinking it is under attack. In prey species, we often use the flight response to our advantage when we want to move the group. However, these animals also will go into the fight response if pushed too hard.

The herd instinct dictates the action of prey animals. There is safety in numbers, and if an individual member of the group is threatened, the rest of the group may come to its aid. For example, when a kid (baby goat) is captured, its usual reaction is to cry out. The kid's cry usually prompts the rest of the herd to come to its defense. This type of behavior is common in groups of pigs, horses, and dogs, as well as goats. Another behavior is to mill around in a circle with the young usually in the center. This confuses the "predator" and with any luck only minor losses to the herd occur. For instance, when cattle are pushed too hard to move into a pen or alley, they will circle around, not wanting to be the one to take the first step "into danger."

Of course, individual animals of the same species will exhibit differences in behavior, as will male and female members of the same species. Female animals in estrus (heat) can become dangerous and aggressive. Female horses (mares) in estrus tend to develop a short temper and do not tolerate other mares around them. The danger here is getting caught between two mares kicking at each other. Female animals with young should also be approached cautiously. All mothers can be very protective if they feel their offspring are being threatened and will defend them to the death if necessary. Depending on the species, sometimes it is best to separate the offspring from the mother before proceeding with any treatment. For example, sows (female pigs) become enraged when they hear the squeals of their piglets, or even piglets that are not their own, and attempt to come to the piglets' aid. The sows may climb over or force their way under corral fences to get to the piglets. In other species, such as horses, young animals should be handled within the mother's sight because the mother is more worried about the physical separation than the handling. If you move a foal out of the mare's sight, both mare and foal will fret vocally and may injure themselves in the attempt to be reunited.

Bulls, boars, and stallions can be very aggressive and extremely dangerous during the mating season. Extreme caution should be observed when handling these animals, especially dairy bulls, whose behavior tends to be unpredictable even under normal circumstances. Some breeds of dogs tend to be more aggressive if intact. A novice should not handle these kinds of animals. If working around these animals makes you uncomfortable, do not attempt to do so, for your own safety and that of the other people involved. Watch, listen, and learn, so that you will be able to handle these animals in time. Remember, animals can sense when you are anxious or afraid.

Some animals are extremely territorial and quickly establish and defend their territory. For example, a cat or dog that is friendly when placed into a hospital cage or run may suddenly become very aggressive when you try to bring it out for examination. Some dogs consider their owners as territory or part of their pack and feel they must guard or protect them. In either case, the animal has territory issues and will defend it against all invaders. One solution is to quickly remove the animal from its perceived territory in a nonaggressive way. The easiest method is to open the door and allow the animal to walk out of the cage or remove the animal from the owner's presence. Obviously this is not appropriate if the room cannot be secured against escape. You should also **not** try this if the animal is aggressively attacking the cage door. However, many animals will calm down and stop being aggressive or protective once removed from their perceived territory.

Some animals have a hierarchy in their pack, group, or herd. These levels of social standing include a dominant animal, after which there are descending levels of status in the pecking order. The position each animal maintains, or tries to maintain, within a group affects behavior. If an animal is removed from the group for even a short time and then returned, that animal may have to fight its way back to its original standing. This can be a dangerous situation for the animal and the human. Members of the animal's group may try to drive it away or in extreme cases even kill it. A person caught between two or more animals fighting can sustain severe injuries. If an individual must be removed from a group, all of the animals should be moved into an enclosure. The individual should be singled out, quickly removed, treated, and returned to the group as promptly as possible. Then the group can be returned to their pen or pasture. The animals that will most likely exhibit this behavior will be dogs, goats, and horses.

Question 2: How can this animal hurt me?

Domestic animals have teeth to bite with; beaks to peck or pinch with; hooves to kick, stomp, and strike with; and claws that can puncture, scratch, and dig. Large animals can use their heads as battering rams, and there is always a chance of being crushed by unrestrained large animals if they should rush a gate or stampede. Take measures to safeguard against these defensive "weapons." Apply muzzles when appropriate, use chutes and stocks for large animals, apply ropes and other restraint equipment as described in later chapters of this book, and always have an escape route in mind should something go wrong.

Animal Safety

Most animals do not quietly submit to forcible restraint. Their resistance may prompt you to hold on a bit tighter. This more forceful restraint may cause the animal to resist even more, eventually resulting in injury to you or the animal.

Each of the various species of animals you may work with has a variety of restraint techniques appropriate for that species. Your job is to match those restraint techniques with the diagnostic or therapeutic procedures being performed and the individual behavior of the animal. This will prevent inadvertent injuries from occurring to you and the animal.

Restraint causes stress in normal, healthy animals, and care should be taken to avoid causing that stress. This is even more important for very young and very old animals. Very young animals have to be treated gently so that their first trips to the veterinarian are not unhappy ones. Similarly, old animals have to be treated gently so that their trips to the veterinarian are not painful. The small bones of young animals and the brittle bones of old animals can be easily broken. The joints on the very young are easily dislocated. In very old animals, manipulation of arthritic joints during restraint can cause pain.

Many of the animals handled by veterinary personnel are sick or injured, and already stressed. Rough handling during restraint may delay recovery or even lead to a premature death. Because pain can precipitate shock, restraint techniques that increase pain in an injured patient may cause death. Pregnant animals are also affected by stress, and complications may arise if they are treated harshly.

After the restraint procedure is completed, the animal should be observed for signs of injury associated with restraint. Unless chemical restraint was used, no ill effects should be noted and the animal should appear as it was before restraint was applied.

Every time you use restraint, you must consider the safety of the animal and the people involved. With some experience, you will be able to foresee problems that could develop during a procedure and take precautions to prevent them. Although the animal's safety is important, human safety must take precedence. If possible, the animal's owner or nonveterinary personnel should not help restrain an animal unless absolutely necessary, because any mishap could have legal repercussions.

RESTRAINT PROCEDURES AND EQUIPMENT

It would be wonderful if our patients cooperated and we did not have to restrain them at all. Unfortunately, physical restraint of an animal is usually unavoidable. However, restraint does not have to be extremely painful or very stressful. Before restraint is applied, you must use good judgment in selecting the proper restraint technique. Do not routinely use a favored technique just because it "always works." You should instead consider the individual and judge what is best to use for that particular procedure.

As stated earlier, animals can be hurt and become psychologically upset if restraint is overly harsh. Restraint techniques must be applied properly and in such a manner as to minimize any pain experienced by the animal. You must have a good working knowledge of animal anatomy, physiology, and behavior to decide what restraint technique to use for a particular procedure.

Equipment

If restraint equipment is to be used during the procedure, examine the equipment and have it ready for use before starting. Nothing is more aggravating or potentially more dangerous than having a piece of equipment fail to function properly or break during the restraint procedure.

The most flexible instruments for restraint are your hands. The hands can soothe and calm an animal and manipulate any part of an animal's body for examination or treatment. However, your hands can also cause fractures or suffocation if used with too much force. You should consider your hands as fragile instruments because they are easily injured by animals. You must protect your hands by learning where and how to grasp animals.

Most restraint instruments are designed for use on a particular species, and many are designed to distract the animal by applying a small amount of pain to a different area of the body than that being worked on. These instruments can cause injury if used incorrectly but are invaluable when used correctly. Uses of many of these instruments are described in later chapters.

Voice

Another important restraint tool is the voice. Almost every domestic animal responds to the tone and pitch of voice used by the handler. Your voice is a powerful instrument, but it can also be a disadvantage if it conveys fear and lack of confidence. Animals are very perceptive of the tone of your voice and body language. If your voice and body language convey that you are anxious or upset, the animal often will become more anxious and upset. Therefore, if you are afraid of an animal, keep quiet and stand still until you can master the fear and continue without arousing the animal's suspicion.

The most common use of the voice is to let the animal know you are approaching it. Undesirable patient behavior, such as striking out or trying to get away, can result if you suddenly appear close to an animal, startling it into a fight-or-flight response. It is wise to begin talking to an animal long before you get close to it. Your voice can also be useful while you are actually handling the animal. When used in combination with manual restraint, quietly speaking to the animal tends to calm the animal and the owner!

Three tones of voice are useful in letting the animal know what is expected: *soothing*, *instructional*, and *commanding*. You should use soft, crooning words in a soothing tone of voice as long as the animal is behaving itself or while you are getting acquainted. Commonly used phrases include "hello," "good, good," "it's okay," "hang in there," and "almost over." You can also use sounds such as a humming or "shhhh." These sounds work well to distract the animal from the procedure being performed. In most instances, any words or sounds can be used, as long as a soothing tone is used. Be careful not to speak too quickly or with a sense of urgency, such as when an injection is about to be given. This alerts the animal that something unpleasant is about to happen, and the animal will tense up or react negatively.

An instructional tone of voice is firm and abrupt and is used when an animal balks or refuses to do what you are asking. Examples include "sit," "no," "move over," and "stop" or "whoa." Be very firm and decisive, and use a lower pitch and speak more loudly than the soothing tone. This tone may also be used to momentarily distract an animal.

A commanding tone of voice is the voice of authority. Some call it the "bad dog voice." Use it when you want the animal to behave and pay attention. It should be very firm and deep, and much louder than the instructional tone. However, do not scream or shout. Screaming indicates a lack of control. The same words can be used as with the instructional tone, but the inflection is different and the consonants are drawn out, as in "Behavvve!" and "Enoughfffff!" You may also have to tug sharply on the leash or lead rope at the same time you issue the command. This will definitely get the animal's attention and can often stop it from acting up.

As with all restraint, the key to success when using your voice is to be gentle but firm and consistent, and not rigid. You give the animal mixed signals if you begin a restraint procedure harshly then ease up on the hold or shout at the animal but then switch to a soothing voice. These mixed signals only confuse the animal, who won't know whether to trust you or be afraid of you.

Chemical restraint involves the use of drugs with effects ranging from sedation to complete immobilization. Sedation or tranquilization can remove fear and anxiety. However, the fight-or-flight response can override the effects, so do not rely heavily on chemical restraint to slow the animal's reactions down. General anesthesia will render the animal completely unconscious. Chemical restraint can be extremely dangerous in the hands of untrained personnel. You must know what drug and what dosage to give to achieve the desired effects. You also need to know how to handle the animal once the drug has been given and how to monitor the animal's heart and respiratory rate. Once sedated or tranquilized, an animal should never be left alone and certainly not left on an examination table unattended! Most times a sedated or tranquilized animal can still walk or crawl and may fall off the examination table, sustaining severe injuries. Remember, a fearful or aggressive animal may become more fearful or aggressive when recovering from anesthesia or sedation, especially if it is in the same situation that caused it to be fearful or aggressive in the first place.

CIRCUMSTANCES FOR RESTRAINT

The ideal setting in which to apply a restraint technique is in a clean, well-lighted, air-conditioned clinic or hospital. But you must also be prepared to perform a restraint technique under less ideal conditions. To do the best job possible, you should keep several considerations in mind while planning and implementing the restraint techniques. These considerations apply to routine circumstances but also should be applied as much as possible to emergency circumstances.

TIME

The best time to apply a restraint technique depends on the species of animal and the type of restraint used. If the procedure involves general anesthesia, the animal should be anesthetized early in the day so it has the remainder of the day to recover. The time of day is also a factor when physically restraining some animals. Some animals are easily handled during their resting periods. Nocturnal animals (active at night) can be handled more easily in

bright light. Conversely, diurnal animals (active during the day) are handled more easily in subdued lighting.

TEMPERATURE

Hot or cold weather conditions can cause problems in restraint. Some species, such as pigs and sheep, become hyperthermic quickly if handled roughly or chased excessively even in slightly warm weather. If possible, plan procedures that require physical restraint for cooler periods of the day. Early morning is often the best time because it is usually cool and the animals can be observed for problems the rest of the day. In emergency situations, various safety measures can help protect the animal from the adverse effects of heat. These include performing the restraint procedure in an area that will remain shady for most of the day, using fans and cool water sprayed on the animal's legs and stomach to cool it, and avoiding heavy restraint techniques when the humidity is higher than 70%.

In cold weather, hypothermia is a concern when animals are to be restrained. Taking advantage of solar heat is wise if a heated barn is not available. This is especially important for animals that have been anesthetized because their body temperatures decrease under anesthesia. Animals anesthetized in a cold environment may become dangerously hypothermic. Care should be taken not to leave them until their body temperatures have returned to normal.

SETTING

The physical environment in which you are working also demands attention. Small animals, such as dogs, cats, rodents, and birds, are usually restrained in an examination room or hospital treatment area. Doors and windows should be securely latched to prevent escape, and countertops should be cleared of excess equipment.

Be sure to consider whether the animal will still be contained if it happens to get away from the restraint. When large animals are to be herded into chutes or corrals, these structures should be inspected before the animals are moved into them. Check for loose boards and protruding nails or splinters. Also check mechanical equipment for proper working condition. If an animal is to be cast, the area should be cleared of objects that could cause injury. Another concern before casting an animal is whether the animal can get its legs caught under fencing or other objects while it is down.

PHEROMONES

Pheromones are chemicals sent outside an animal's body that signal other animals. There are commercially available pheromones that can be purchased for dogs and cats to help alleviate stress. These can be used in a clinical setting as aerosols or applied directly to restraint devices.

PERSONNEL

Veterinarians, veterinary technicians, and veterinary assistants are capable of restraining animals. The person selected to apply the restraint depends on the procedure to be done, help available, and circumstances involved. Owners should **never** be asked to restrain their animals for a procedure. They do not understand the complexities of restraint nor what it will take to keep an animal under control for the duration of the procedure. Many lawsuits have been filed by owners who have been hurt while restraining their animals, and many juries have found the veterinarians who were involved negligent.

PLANNING

As part of the veterinary team, technicians must ensure that animals under their care are treated in the best manner possible. This means that every restraint procedure must be preceded by thorough planning to ensure the safety of everyone involved. You must know which restraint techniques work well on the various types of animals. When a combination of procedures will be used, you must plan the sequence of restraint techniques so that you can switch from one to another without having to stop and decide on the next step. Also, the animal's temperament may change as the procedure is carried out, so you should start with the least amount of restraint possible and work into more restrictive techniques as needed.

DURATION

The duration of the restraint technique must also be taken into consideration. You should not initiate a restraint technique until everyone is ready to do his or her part of the procedure. An animal held in an unnatural position for even a short period may begin to struggle, making the procedure stressful for you and the animal.

The restraint technique should be applied quickly and confidently. Serious injuries can result if it is applied sloppily or incorrectly. You must know how to restrain the animal before you apply any restraint. If you are unsure of how to apply a specific type of restraint, it should not be attempted.

COMPLICATIONS

Regardless of how well a restraint technique is planned, unpredicted events may cause problems. By anticipating problems, you can better deal with them if and when they occur. Some animals do not respond to gentle words and caresses. Drastic measures must be taken to control these animals, such as chemical restraint. The main point to remember in these situations is not to lose your temper. If you become angry, you decrease the likelihood that the animal will cooperate. Animals can readily sense your anger and frustration and are likely to become more agitated.

As you review the following chapters, bear in mind that you must always strive to use the minimum amount of restraint necessary to complete a procedure. This does not mean that you should apply no restraint, as that could result in injury. Rather, begin with a gentle hand and a reassuring voice and progressively apply more restraint as needed.

SUGGESTED READINGS

Fowler ME: *Restraint and handling of wild and domestic animals*, Ames, IA, 1978, Iowa State University Press.

Grandin T: *Genetics and behavior of domestic animals*, San Diego, 1998, Academic Press.

Grandin T: *Animals make us human*, Boston, 2010, Houghton Mifflin Harcourt.

Leahy JR, Barrow P: *Restraint of animals*, Ithaca, NY, 1953, Cornell Campus Store.

Sonsthagen TF: *Restraint of domestic animals*, St. Louis, 1991, Mosby.

Todd-Jenkins K, Dugan B, Remsburg DW, Montgomery C: Restraint and handling of animals. In *McCurnin's clinical textbook for veterinary technicians*, ed 8, Philadelphia, 2014, Saunders.

Yin S: *Low stress handling, restraint and behavior modification of dogs and cats: techniques for developing patients who love their visits*, Davis, CA, 2009, CattleDog Publishing.

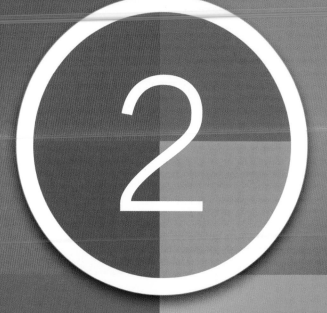

Knot Tying

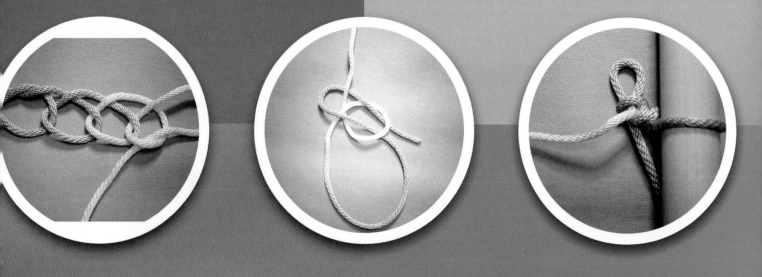

Restraining animals often requires the use of ropes and knots to secure the animals to objects or to immobilize them. It is therefore important that you learn how to tie the basic knots and hitches used to restrain animals. In addition, many circumstances in everyday life require knowledge of tying a secure knot.

TERMINOLOGY

Knots are an "intertwining of one or two ropes in which the pressure of the standing part of the rope alone prevents the end from slipping." Hitches are a "temporary fastening of a rope to a hook, post, or other object, with the rope arranged so that the standing part forces the end against the object with sufficient pressure to prevent slipping."

The *standing part* of the rope is the longer end of the rope or the end attached to the animal. The *end* is the short end of the rope or the end that you can freely move about. A *bight* is a sharp bend in the rope (Fig. 2-1).

A *loop* or *half hitch* is a complete circle formed in the rope. A loop can open toward you (Fig. 2-2, *A*) or away from you (Fig. 2-2, *B*). Careful attention to how a loop opens ensures that your knots or hitches will be successful.

A *throw* is when one rope is wrapped around another to make part of a knot (Fig. 2-3). An *overhand knot* is the base knot for a number of different knots (Fig. 2-4). To form an overhand knot, make a half hitch, then bring the end through the resulting loop.

EQUIPMENT MAINTENANCE

It is important to inspect the ropes for tears or stressed points in the strands, dirt, and kinks. These weaken the rope, causing it to give way under stress. If the rope is soiled, wash it in warm water. Avoid using detergents

or soaps because they can deteriorate the rope's fibers, weakening the rope. After you have cleaned the rope, allow it to dry thoroughly before putting it away so that it does not become moldy. Keep in mind that your rope needs to be in good working order for all restraint situations, including emergencies. Your life and the animal's life depend on it.

When storing ropes, coil or secure them properly to prevent kinks or twists. "Hanking" is one method that

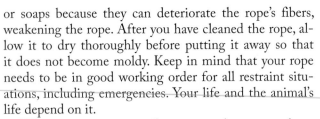

FIG. 2-2

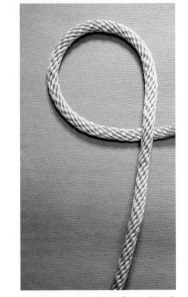

A loop or half hitch is a complete circle formed in the rope. A loop can open toward you (**A**).

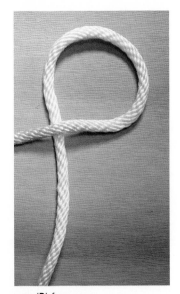

A loop can move away (**B**) from you.

FIG. 2-1

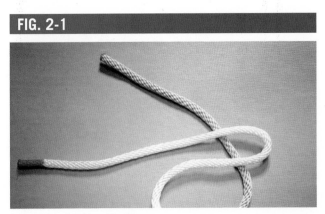

A bight is a sharp bend in the rope.

FIG. 2-3

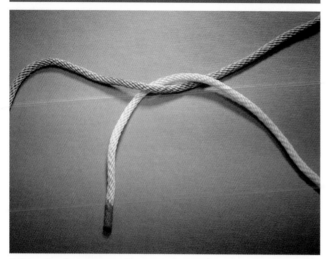

A throw is when one rope is wrapped around another to make part of a knot.

FIG. 2-4

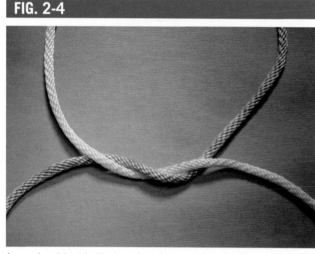

An overhand knot is the base knot for a number of different knots. You form one by making a half hitch and then bringing the end through the resulting loop.

FIG. 2-5

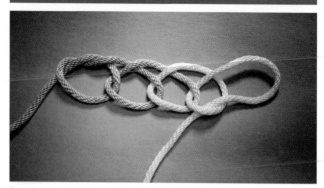

Stored ropes should be properly coiled or secured to prevent kinks or twists. "Hanking" is one method that works well on long lengths of rope and electrical cords.

FIG. 2-6

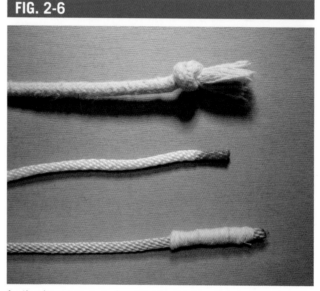

Another important part of maintaining equipment is to prevent unraveling or fraying of the ends of the rope. One of the easiest methods is called "whipping."

works well on long lengths of rope and electrical cords (Fig. 2-5). Start by making a loop that opens toward you at one end of the rope. Hold the loop in place with your left hand. With your right hand, reach through the loop and grasp the standing portion of the rope and pull a bight through the loop. This bight now becomes the next loop. Continue in this manner until the rope is chain crocheted to the opposite end. To fasten the rope after reaching the opposite end, simply pass the end through the last loop you made and tighten. To unravel the rope, remove the end from the last loop you made and pull; it should unravel easily. If not, you probably have the wrong end.

Another important part of maintaining equipment is to prevent the ends of the rope from unraveling or fraying. The four easiest methods are (1) tying a simple overhand knot close to both ends, (2) melting the ends (nylon ropes) with a match or lighter, (3) coating them with a stop-fraying product, or (4) whipping (Fig. 2-6).

FIG. 2-7

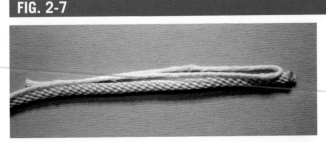

A To whip a rope, lay about 4 inches of the smaller cord lengthwise near the tip of the rope. Make a bight close to the end of the rope, with the smaller cord running down so that you have two strands, each 4 inches long.

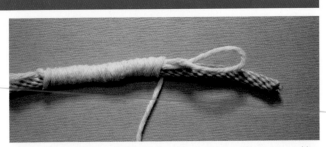

B Start to wrap the cord around the two strands and the rope, making sure to leave a small tag below the wrapped strands.

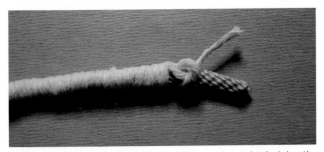

C Once you have covered both strands of the cord completely, bring the end of the cord through the bight.

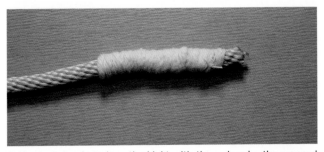

D The last step is to bury the bight with the end under the wrapped strands of rope. Do this by pulling on the tag that was left uncovered.

Whipping is done with a cord of a smaller diameter than the rope being whipped. Begin about 1 to 1½ inches away from the end of the rope to prevent the whipping from falling off the end. Lay about 4 inches of the smaller cord lengthwise near the tip of the rope. Make a bight close to the end of the rope, with the smaller cord running down so you have two strands, each 4 inches long (Fig. 2-7, *A*). Start to wrap the cord around the two strands and the rope, making sure to leave a small tag below the wrapped strands (Fig. 2-7, *B*). Once you have covered both strands of the cord completely, bring the end of the cord through the bight (Fig. 2-7, *C*). The last step is to bury the bight with the end under the wrapped strands of rope. Do this by pulling on the tag left uncovered (Fig. 2-7, *D*). Clip the tag off close to the wrap to finish the whipping process.

TYPES OF KNOTS

SQUARE KNOT

The square knot is used to secure the ends of two ropes together or to form a nonslipping noose. A nonslipping knot is one that will not come untied or tighten if pressure is applied to both ends. This knot is commonly used to secure sutures. An easy way to remember how to tie a square knot is to use the saying "right over left (Fig. 2-8, *A*), left over right (Fig. 2-8, *B*)." The same rope used to make the first throw should be used to make the second throw. A properly tied square knot forms what looks like two intertwined loops (Fig. 2-8, *C*) and is easily untied when the opposite ends are pushed together (Fig. 2-8, *D*).

FIG. 2-8

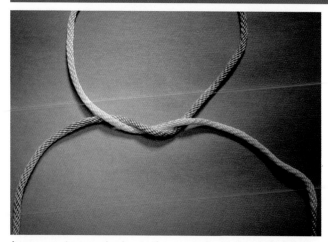

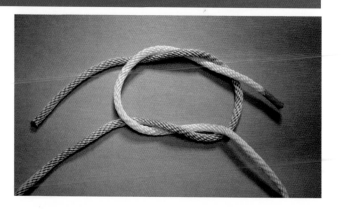

An easy way to remember how to tie a square knot is to use the following saying: "right over left (**A**), left over right (**B**)."

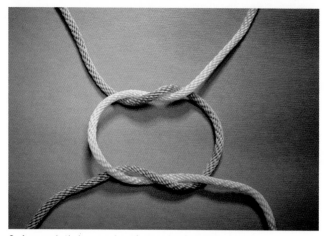

C A properly tied square knot forms what looks like two intertwined loops.

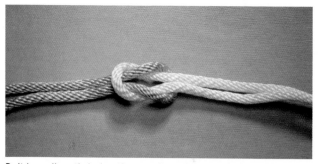

D It is easily untied when the opposite ends are pushed together.

SURGEON'S KNOT

The surgeon's knot is used when a package or load cannot be secured because the first throw loosens while the second throw is being placed. This occurs in surgery when the skin is tight and will not stay closed as the surgeon tries to make the next throw.

The surgeon's knot starts with two throws on the first half of the knot (Fig. 2-9). This keeps the knot from slipping while you place a square knot on top of the throws. As in the square knot, it is important to use the same end that made the first throw to continue making the next two. The surgeon's knot should always have a square knot on top to keep it secure.

FIG. 2-9

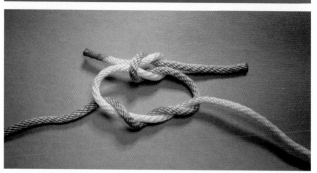

The surgeon's knot starts with two throws on the first half of the knot. This keeps the knot from slipping while you place a square knot on top of the throws.

FIG. 2-10

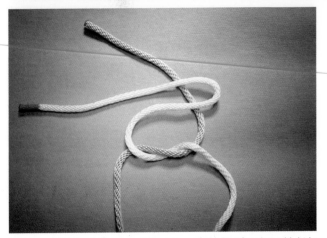

A For a reefer's knot, the second throw is made by first forming a bight in the left-hand rope and tightening the knot with the bight in place.

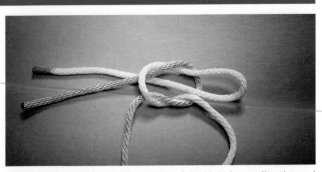

B To tighten this knot, pull the middle of the bight in one direction and the ends in the opposite direction.

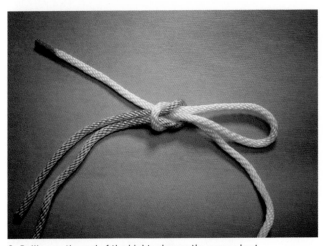

C Pulling on the end of the bight releases the square knot.

REEFER'S KNOT (SINGLE BOW KNOT)

The reefer's knot allows you to tie a nonslipping, quick-release knot. The reefer's knot is the same as the square knot, with one exception. You make the second throw by first forming a bight in the left-hand rope (Fig. 2-10, *A*) and tightening the knot with the bight in place. To tighten this knot, pull the middle of the bight in one direction and the other end in the opposite direction (Fig. 2-10, *B*). Pulling on the end of the bight will release the square knot (Fig. 2-10, *C*).

TOMFOOL KNOT (DOUBLE BOW KNOT)

The tomfool knot is another variant of the square knot, which is used to bind two limbs together. To make the tomfool knot, find the center of the rope, make a loop so

that it opens toward you, and hold the loop in your left hand. Make a second loop that opens away from you and hold it in your right hand (Fig. 2-11, *A*). Move the two loops so that the right one is underneath and halfway across the left (Fig. 2-11, *B*). Wrap your index finger around the side of the left-hand loop as your index finger and middle fingers grasp the side of the right-hand loop. Slide the right side up through the left loop and the left side down through the right loop (Fig. 2-11, *C*). The result is two adjustable loops that open when you pull on the loops themselves and close when you pull on the ends (Fig. 2-11, *D*). You can easily untie a properly tied tomfool knot by pulling on the ends of the rope. To secure the knot more firmly, place a square knot or reefer's knot on top of the resulting knot to hold the loops in the desired size.

FIG. 2-11

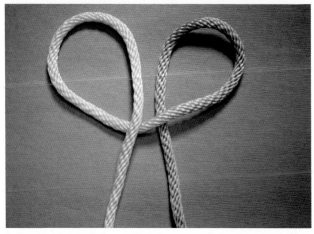

A To make the tomfool knot, find the center of the rope, make a loop so that it opens toward you, and hold the loop in your left hand. Make a second loop that opens away from you and hold it in your right hand.

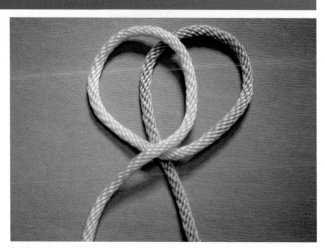

B Move the two loops so the right one is underneath and halfway across the left.

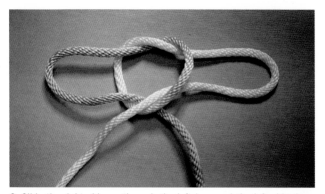

C Slide the right side up through the left loop and the left side down through the right loop.

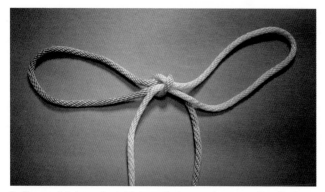

D The result is two adjustable loops that open when you pull on the loops themselves and close when you pull on the ends.

HALTER TIE (QUICK-RELEASE KNOT)

The halter tie is a quick-release knot that should always be used when securing an animal to an immovable object. If the animal becomes entangled in the rope, is frightened, or goes down for any reason, a quick pull on the end of the rope releases the animal so that it is not injured while struggling. Once you learn the basic knot, practice using it on a real horse or cow attached to the standing part of your rope, or have someone hold the standing part. Be sure to practice the knot by tying the animal with it standing on your left and then on your right as well as on horizontal and vertical bars. It seems to throw people when they actually have to use the knot!

To tie the halter knot, pass the end of the rope around the post or rail, and make a loop on the end that opens toward you, fairly close to the post. Lay the loop on the top of the standing part of the rope, holding onto the loop and the standing part with your left hand (Fig. 2-12, *A*). Make a bight slightly farther down on the end and pass it behind the standing part of the rope and up through the loop (Fig. 2-12, *B*). Pull only the bight through the loop, leaving the protruding end to be used to loosen the knot. Slide the knot along the standing part to place the knot close to the post or rail (Fig. 2-12, *C*). To be sure it is a quick-release knot, pull on the end of the rope; the knot should untie without any resistance.

When tying an animal to an immovable object, always keep the rope short enough and high enough so the animal cannot step over the rope or become entangled in it. To keep an animal from releasing itself by pulling on the end, put the end through the loop. Note that you must pull the end back out of the loop to release the knot.

FIG. 2-12

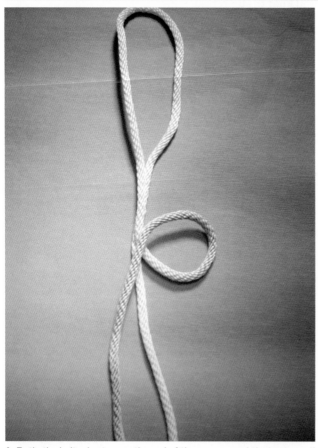

A To tie the halter knot, pass the end of the rope around the post or rail and make a loop on the end that opens toward you, fairly close to the post. Lay the loop on the top of the standing part of the rope, holding onto the loop and the standing part with your left hand.

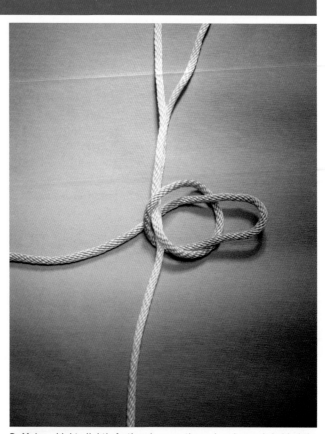

B Make a bight slightly farther down on the end and pass it behind the standing part of the rope and up through the loop.

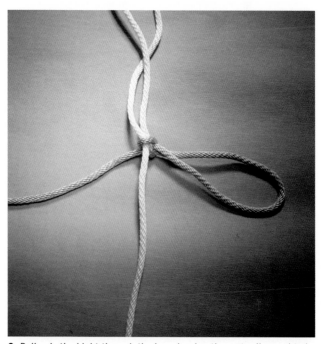

C Pull only the bight through the loop, leaving the protruding end to be used to loosen the knot. Slide the knot along the standing part to place the knot close to the post or rail.

SHEET BEND

The sheet bend is used to tie two ropes of different sizes securely together. Make a bight in the larger rope and run the end of the smaller rope through the center of the bight (Fig. 2-13, *A*), then back around behind the two parts of the bight in the larger rope (Fig. 2-13, *B*). Bring it under the smaller cord in the center (Fig. 2-13, *C*) and tighten by pulling on the end of the smaller cord (Fig. 2-13, *D*).

This knot can be used as a tail tie on a horse or cow. When using it on the tail, be sure to apply the rope beyond the last coccygeal vertebra. The hair on the tail is the larger "rope"; hold it so the hair is all together and forms the bight. When tightening the knot, pull on the end of the small rope until the knot is closed, then use the standing part to tighten it. Pulling only on the end will cause the knot to slip off the tail.

BOWLINE

There are many variations of the bowline knot. The principle is to make a nonslip noose that will not tighten. The resulting noose is safe to place around an animal's neck and is easy to untie, no matter how tight the knot is pulled. To start the knot, make a loop so that it opens away from you in the standing part of the rope (Fig. 2-14, *A*). Bring the end of the rope through the loop from the back or bottom (Fig. 2-14, *B*) and then pass the end around the standing part of the rope

---

FIG. 2-13

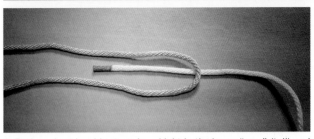

A To tie a sheet bend knot, make a bight in the larger "rope" (tail) and run the end of the smaller rope through the center of the bight.

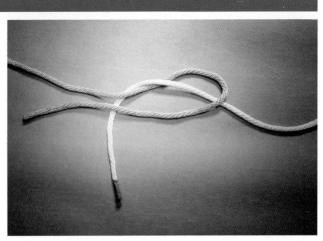

B Then run the end of the smaller rope back behind the two parts of the bight in the larger "rope" (tail).

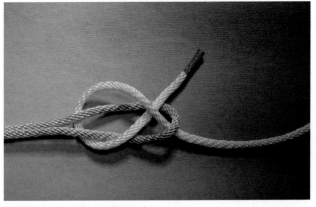

C Bring it under the smaller cord.

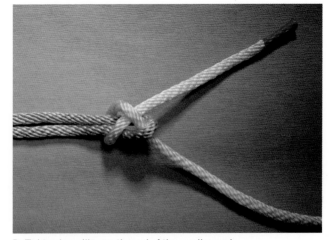

D Tighten by pulling on the end of the smaller cord.

FIG. 2-14

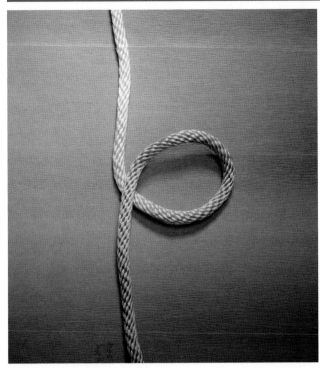

A To start the bowline knot, make a loop so that it opens away from you in the standing part of the rope.

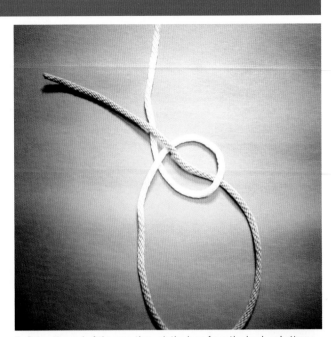

B Bring the end of the rope through the loop from the back or bottom.

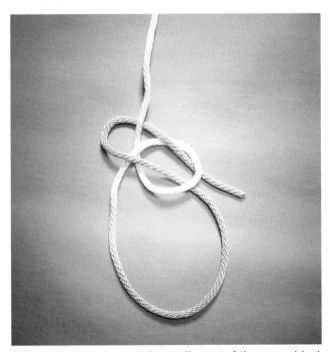

C Then pass the end around the standing part of the rope and back through the loop, this time from the front or top.

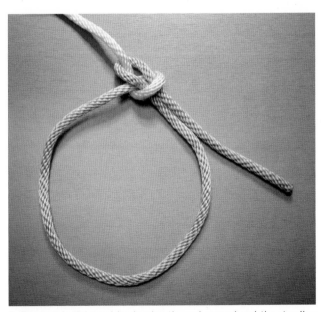

D The knot is tightened by drawing the end upward and the standing part downward.

and back through the loop again, this time from the front or top (Fig. 2-14, *C*). Tighten the knot by drawing the end upward and the standing part downward (Fig. 2-14, *D*).

The following saying can help you remember how to tie this knot. The end of the rope is referred to as the "rabbit," and the standing part is referred to as the "tree." After making the loop, "the rabbit comes out of its hole, goes around behind the tree, and back into its hole."

BOWLINE ON THE BIGHT

This is a good knot for placing a rope around an animal's neck and securing the legs with the same rope. The noose is nonslipping and the ends are of equal length. Because the knot does not tighten, because it is a bowline, it is also easy to untie. Double the rope in half and tie an overhand knot, leaving a large loop (Fig. 2-15, *A*). Reach through the bight with your right hand and grasp the bottom of the overhand knot. With your left hand, grasp the middle of the bight (Fig. 2-15, *B*, step 1) and, while moving your right hand back and up, pull the bight to the left until your right hand is all the way through the bight (Fig. 2-15, *B*, steps 2 and 3). Release the bight with your left hand but continue to hold onto the loop with your right hand. With both hands, pull the two sides of the loop in opposite directions to tighten the knot (Fig. 2-15, *C*). If you slide the knot down to the bight instead of pulling on both sides of the loop, the resulting knot is a sliding noose that is very dangerous around an animal's neck. The finished knot leaves you a nonslipping noose and ends of equal length (Fig. 2-15, *D*).

FIG. 2-15

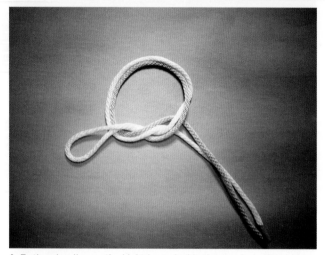

A To tie a bowline on the bight knot, double the rope in half and tie an overhand knot, leaving a large loop.

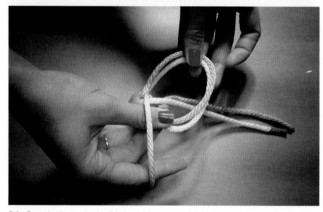

B1 Reach through the bight with your right hand and grasp the bottom of the overhand knot. With your left hand, grasp the middle of the bight.

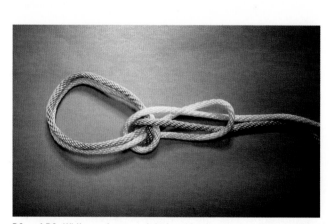

B2 and B3 While moving your right hand back and up, pull the bight to the left until your right hand is all the way through the bight.

(**Figure 2-15,** continued on following page)

FIG. 2-15 cont.

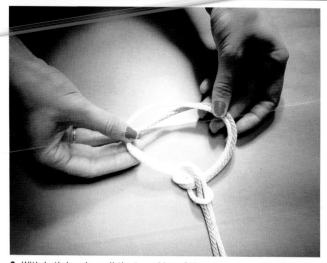

C With both hands, pull the two sides of the loop in opposite directions to tighten the knot.

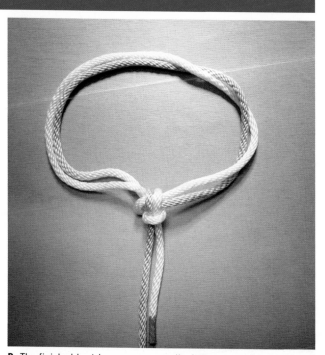

D The finished knot leaves you a nonslipping noose and ends of equal length.

FIG. 2-16

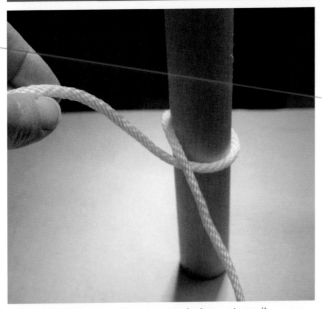

A To tie a half hitch, pass the rope around a leg, post, or rail.

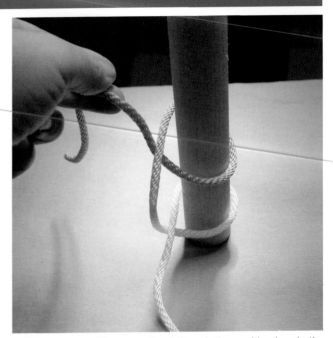

B The next pass will go around and through the resulting loop in the standing part.

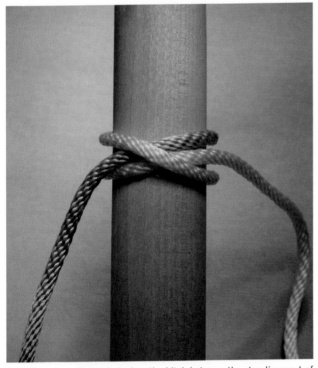

C Pulling up on the end pinches the hitch between the standing part of the rope and the post.

HALF HITCH

The half hitch is a loop that can either be opened toward or away from you, depending on the requirements of the knot. The half hitch is good as a temporary fastening if steady pressure is going to be applied to the rope, such as when tying an animal to a surgery table.

Two half hitches are needed if attaching a rope to a post. Start by making a half hitch by passing the rope around a leg, post, or rail (Fig. 2-16, *A*), with the next pass going around and through the resulting loop in the standing part (Fig. 2-16, *B*). Pulling up on the end pinches the hitch between the standing part of the rope and the post (Fig. 2-16, *C*). Both ends are free to be used for whatever reason. The hitch will not come undone even when one end is used and the other is not.

FIG. 2-17

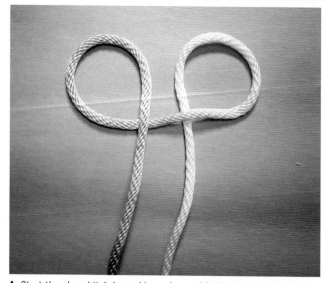

A Start the clove hitch by making a loop, with the loop opening toward you and another loop facing away from you.

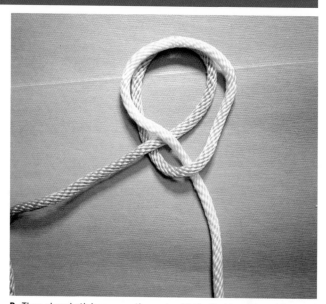

B Then place both loops over the post, with the first loop placed first and the second placed directly on top of that.

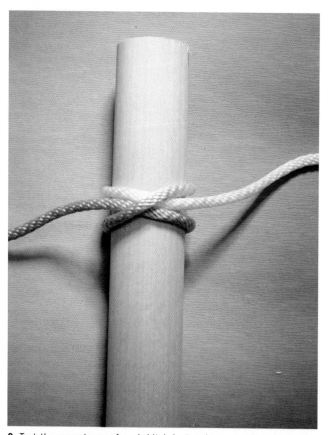

C Test the correctness of each hitch by tugging on each end one at a time and then together.

CLOVE HITCH

The clove hitch, which is the same as two half hitches stacked on one another, is the fastest, easiest, and most convenient way to secure a rope to a vertical bar. It can be used in the middle of the rope or at the ends. You can apply tension to one or both ends of the rope, and the hitch will not slip.

Start the clove hitch by making a loop with the loop opening toward you and another loop facing away from you (Fig. 2-17, *A*). This initial step is similar to that used for the tomfool knot. Then place both loops over the post, with the loop opening toward you placed on first and the second directly on top of that (Fig. 2-17, *B*). Test the correctness of each hitch by tugging on each end one at a time and then together (Fig. 2-17, *C*). If the rope slips, the loops were made incorrectly. Try again by turning one of the loops in the opposite direction.

FIG. 2-18

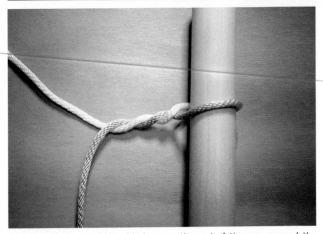

A To secure the snubbing hitch, wrap the end of the rope around the standing part two or more times.

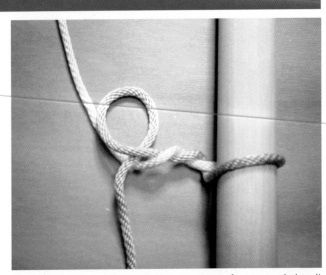

B On the last wrap, make a loop that opens away from you and place it on top of the standing part.

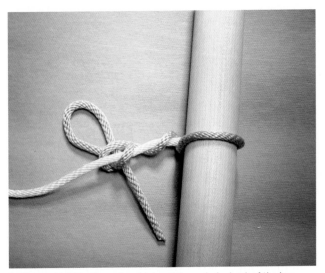

C Make a bight in the end and bring it through the back of the loop.

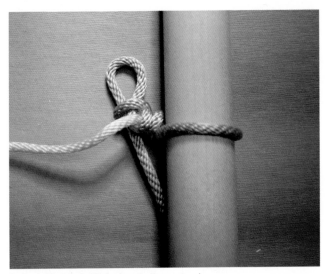

D Push the whole hitch close to the post or brace.

SNUBBING HITCH

The snubbing hitch is used to hold an animal to a post by either a halter rope or nose lead (see Chapter 5, Restraint of Cattle). The snubbing hitch allows slack to be taken up or given, and it can be secured to allow the handler to perform other duties.

The snubbing hitch unsecured is simply a half hitch placed around a post or brace on a chute. To secure the hitch, simply wrap the end of the rope around the standing part two or more times (Fig. 2-18, *A*). On the last wrap, proceed to tie a halter tie; make a loop (Fig. 2-18, *B*) that opens away from you and place it on top of the standing part. Make a bight in the end and bring it through the back of the loop (Fig. 2-18, *C*). Push the whole hitch close to the post or brace (Fig. 2-18, *D*). You can give the rope slack by pulling down on the end releasing the bight. This action will make the hitch unsecure and the handler will have to reapply the bight or hang onto the rope.

3

Restraint of Cats

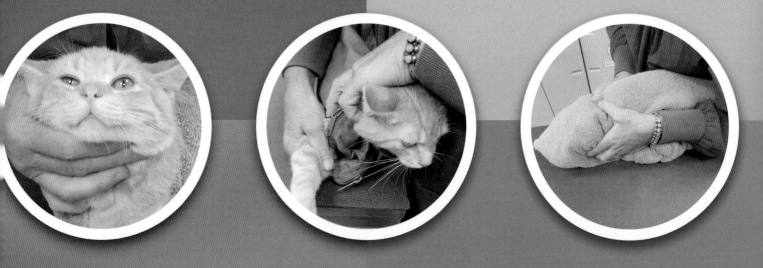

BEHAVIOR

Despite attempts to domesticate cats, they retain much of their instinctive behavior as predators. Cats establish territories quickly and will defend those territories with a very well-equipped arsenal. They object to being held "captive" (i.e., restraint procedures) for extended lengths of time and seem to have good memories for bad experiences. Cats have always relied on their speed, caution, needle-sharp teeth, and dagger-like claws for survival. Our domestic friends have no problem using these defensive weapons when their territory is invaded or when they feel threatened, which can happen with improper restraint techniques.

You cannot establish dominance over a cat as with a dog. You have to meet the cat on its own terms. A greeting between two cats consists of slowly approaching each other; if they like what they see and smell, they will move closer and allow a caress. If they do not like what they see and smell, cats usually lean back, put their ears down, and may vocalize with a hiss or low growl. This warns the other cat off, and the weaker of the two will retreat. If neither of the cats backs down, one or the other will growl louder and "punch" with its front leg to exert a bit more force. This may go on for quite a while before one of the two retreats; if neither retreats, a wholesale fight may ensue.

Knowing this behavior enables veterinary professionals to approach a cat in the veterinary clinic and interpret how it is going to react. If you extend curled fingers for the cat to sniff (and it likes what it smells) and you talk to it in a low soothing voice, most cats will respond in a positive manner. The cat will allow you to caress it and pick it up or hold it. Continue petting, and look for the "itchy" spot at the base of the cat's tail or behind its ears continue to talk to it while gently placing it into a restraint hold. This builds trust with the cat and, if you follow the golden rule of *using minimal restraint at all times,* you will still have a friend at the end of the procedure.

As mentioned previously, not all cats will like what they see, smell, or hear and will try to warn you off. Pay attention to the cat's body language. If its ears are pulled back, if it is leaning away from you, vocalizing, and batting at you, you should recognize these as signals of an unhappy or aggressive cat. In addition, cats flick their tails when unhappy, unlike dogs. Unfortunately, you cannot just back off and leave these cats alone. Their owners would not be too happy with you if you announced that the cat did not want its vaccinations that day! Therefore, you must employ other means of handling the cat. Towel wraps, cat restraint bags, and sometimes even chemical restraint may be necessary with these patients. These techniques are discussed later in this chapter.

You will also want to watch your friendly cat; if it starts to feel threatened it will let you know with the same signals. Your actions at this point will determine whether the cat will allow you to finish the procedure or not. You can divert the cat with distraction techniques—tightening and loosening your hold is one technique to distract the cat—and encourage the person doing the procedure to hurry. If the cat loses its composure and is escaping from your restraint hold, you need to alert the person doing the procedure that you are losing your grip and to finish quickly or to back away. Try not to allow the cat to escape because a cat that has "escaped" once from a hold will fight more vigorously during the next hold.

PRECAUTIONS FOR RESTRAINING CATS

Follow these important rules when handling cats:
1. Make sure all doors, windows, and cabinets are closed because an escaped cat can squeeze through amazingly small openings.
2. Remove all bottles and equipment from the examination table before starting the procedure. Murphy's law dictates that the most expensive piece of equipment or medication will be knocked off the examination table by a struggling cat.
3. Use *minimal* restraint to start a procedure and only tighten your hold as necessary. Applying medium or maximum restraint at the onset will often upset the cat and it will fight to get away. This does not mean that you should not maintain a secure hold; you can maintain control by holding gently but be ready to tighten the hold if the cat's temperament starts to change.
4. Don't treat all cats the same. Read the cat's body language; if it is a gentle cat, handle it gently. Use towels, cat bags, gauntlets, and chemical restraint as necessary on those cats that require more restraint.
5. Use distraction techniques. A cat's attention can be diverted while you perform unpleasant procedures. Timing is of the utmost importance. Begin the diversion just as you start the procedure. Otherwise you may convey anxiety to the cat by increasing the strength of your diversion just as the injection is being given or as a painful procedure begins. Techniques that seem to work well include making a funny noise (be careful with this one; you don't want to scare the cat), vigorously scratching the cat's ears or under its chin, gently tapping its face, blowing on its nose, or wiggling its legs.
6. Above all, don't lose your temper. Remember that cats don't like to be held tightly. It is their nature to fight being "captured." If you lose your temper,

chances are you will tighten your hold to punish an uncooperative cat; the result is that someone will probably get hurt—either the cat (physically or psychologically), the person doing the procedure, or you!

GUIDELINES FOR RESTRAINING CATS

Cats have a fine arsenal of weapons that can cause a great deal of damage to the person restraining them. The key is to accomplish the procedure without being bitten or scratched. Here are some tips to keep you safe and the cat unharmed.

RESTRAINING THE HEAD

There are a number of ways to hold a cat's head without choking the cat. The first method is scruffing, which looks uncomfortable for the cat, but actually has a calming influence. Think of a queen moving her kittens. She picks each one up by the scruff and carries it to its new home. The kitten's response is to go limp, draw its hind feet up, and tuck its tail so that it is not stepped on. This response persists to some degree in the adult cat, which may be thinking, "Mamma is back, and I must be cooperative." When scruffing, be sure to remove the cat's collar first; then, using your dominant hand, grasp as much loose skin as possible behind the head and neck. The procedure you are going to perform dictates the direction of your thumb (Fig. 3-1). This technique allows you to hold the cat's head securely

without making it feel trapped. Some clients may object to this hold, so be ready to move on to the next way of securing the cat's head.

A second technique is to cup the head. Come from the side so that your thumb is on top of the cat's head and your fingers reach under its chin and rest across the mandibles (Fig. 3-2, *A*). You should be able to do this with both right and left hands (Fig. 3-2, *B*). Make sure your fingers stay on its mandibles or the cat will feel like you are choking it and will struggle to get away.

FIG. 3-2

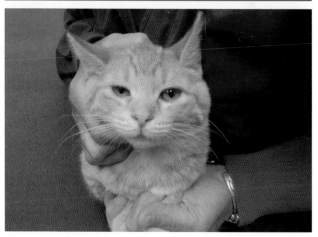

A Come from the side of the head so that your thumb is on top of the head and your fingers reach under the chin and rest across the mandibles.

FIG. 3-1

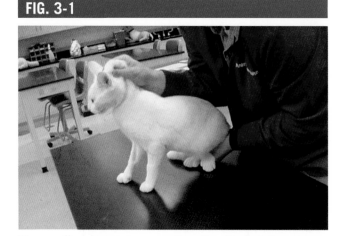

When scruffing, be sure to remove the cat's collar first, then use your dominant hand to grasp as much loose skin as possible behind the head and neck.

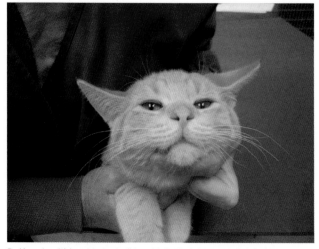

B You should be able to do this with both right and left hands.

FIG. 3-3

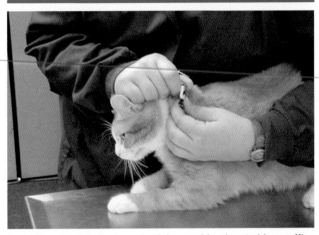

A Set the cat on the table, maintaining good head control by scruffing the cat including the collar. Keep your arm along the cat's body and snug it close to your body.

FIG. 3-4

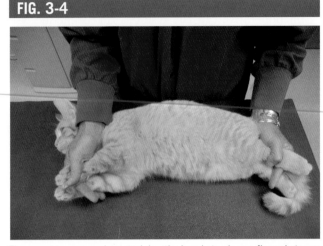

The secret to success in restraining the legs is to place a finger between the legs as you grip them.

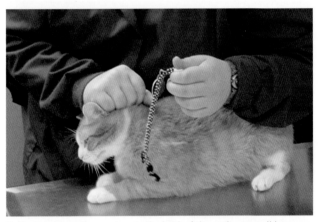

B Unclasp the collar as close to the back of the neck as possible.

REMOVING A COLLAR

Our patients often come in with collars around their necks. A collar can interfere with a number of procedures, so it is important to take it off and keep track of it so that you can put it back on after you are done. Set the cat on the table and maintain good head control by scruffing the cat including the collar. Keep your arm along the cat's body and snug it close to your body (Fig. 3-3, *A*). Unclasp the collar as close to the back of the cat's neck as possible. This keeps your hand away from the cat's mouth and front claws. Place the collar in your pocket so you can easily retrieve it (Fig. 3-3, *B*).

RESTRAINING THE LEGS

The secret to success in restraining a cat's legs in lateral recumbency is to place your finger between the legs as you grip them above the paws (Fig. 3-4). This prevents the cat's legs from slipping between your hands, and you do not have to squeeze as hard to hold onto the legs. When the cat is in a sitting position and you need to grip the front legs higher, with the cat's elbows seated in the palm of your hand, place a finger in between the legs.

REMOVING FROM CAGE OR CARRIER

Earlier we said that cats are very territorial. When placed into a cage or carrier, a cat may establish the enclosure as its territory. The cat will defend its territory if the territory is invaded by a human or another animal. Even an animal being carried past a cat's kennel door may provoke defensive behavior that is often mistaken for aggression. The best way to remove that cat from its cage or carrier is to allow it to move out of its territory on its own. Close all exterior room openings first, then open the cage or carrier door and allow the cat to step out. If this does not work after a reasonable amount of time, tip the carrier a bit or step away from the cage door. Cats can hardly resist the invitation to explore. If the cat still will not exit the cage or carrier, assess the cat's behavior. If it is just scared and not aggressive, you will have to reach in the carrier door or detach the top of the carrier to retrieve the cat. With your right hand, get ready to open the cage. With your left hand, distract the cat to move it away from the opening door (Fig. 3-5, *A*). With one quick motion, open the cage door with your left hand and reach in to scruff the cat with your right hand (Fig. 3-5, *B*). Reach in with your left hand and support the cat's abdomen (Fig. 3-5, *C*). Lift the cat out, pinning it to your right hip with your forearm and elbow. Be sure to support its body. With the cat pinned to your right hip and holding the scruff with your right hand, shut the cage door with your left hand (Fig. 3-5, *D*).

FIG. 3-5

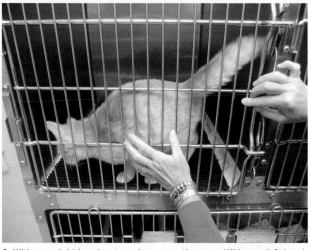

A With your right hand, get ready to open the cage. With your left hand, distract the cat to move it away from the opening door.

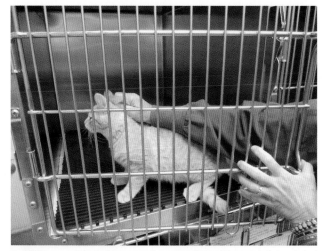

B With one quick motion, open the cage door with your left hand and reach in to scruff the cat with your right hand.

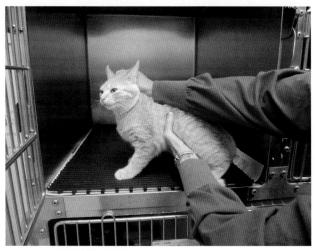

C Reach in with your left hand and support the cat's abdomen.

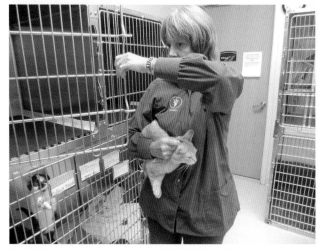

D Lift the cat out, pinning it to your right hip with your forearm and elbow. With the cat on your right hip, hold the scruff with your right hand and shut the cage door with your left hand.

(**Figure 3-5,** continued on following page)

FIG. 3-5 cont.

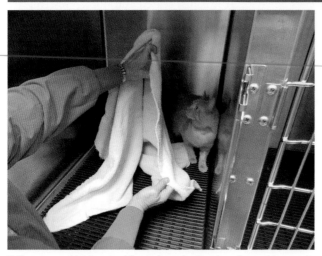

E To remove a frightened cat from a kennel, a towel can be used to cover it.

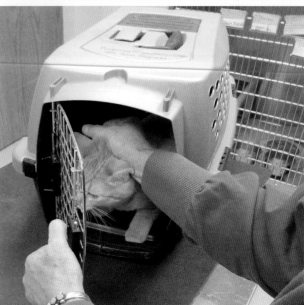

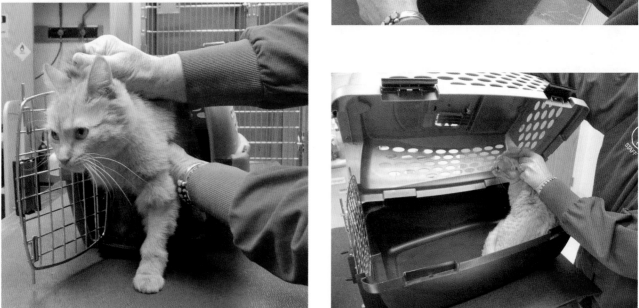

F-H Open the carrier door and determine whether you can easily reach in without threatening the cat. If the cat appears frightened, it is often safer to disassemble the carrier.

A frightened or threatening cat can be removed from a kennel by throwing a towel over it (Fig. 3-5, *E*). Refer to Fig. 3-22 for working with a cat in a full body towel.

Removing a cat from a carrier can be threatening to the cat. If the cat approaches the door, opening the door and quickly scruffing the cat may be successful. Be sure to support the cat's body as you remove it from the carrier so it does not feel as if it is falling (Fig. 3-5, *F* and *G*). Frightened cats respond better to being removed from the carrier if you disassemble the carrier (Fig. 3-5, *H*). It may be necessary to throw a towel over the cat once the carrier is disassembled.

FIG. 3-6

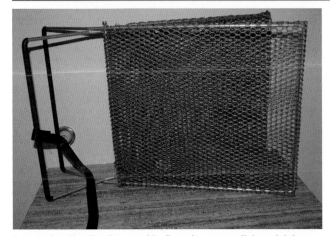

A A device like the "easy-nabber" works very well in subduing an aggressive cat.

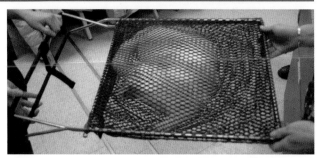

B You can transport the cat to an examination table or wherever you need to take it.

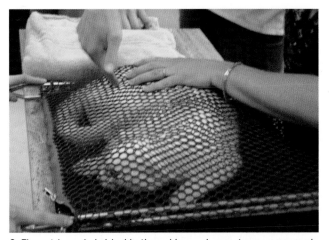

C The cat is encircled inside the nabber and cannot move very much, so intramuscular or subcutaneous injections can be given through the netting.

If you cannot get a hand on the cat, then you will need to use restraint equipment. You can throw a towel over the cat and then scoop it out of the cage and move it to an examination table. A device like the "easy-nabber" works well in subduing an aggressive cat so that it may be given a sedative or tranquilizer without fear that it will bite or scratch the veterinary professional (Fig. 3-6, *A*). You can transport the cat to an examination table or wherever you need to go with it (Fig. 3-6, *B*). The cat is encircled inside the nabber and cannot move much, so intramuscular (IM) or subcutaneous (SQ) injections can be given through the netting (Fig. 3-6, *C*). The netting has a zipper so it can be removed for cleaning.

FIG. 3-7

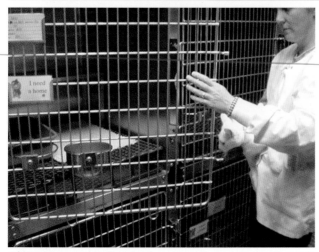

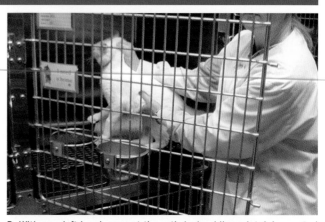

A With the cat on your right hip and your right hand holding the scruff, open the cage door with your left hand.

B With your left hand, support the cat's body while maintaining control of its head with your right hand and lift the cat toward the rear of the cage.

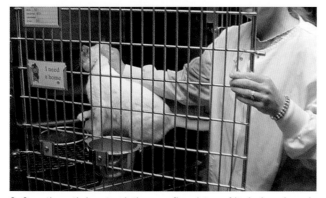

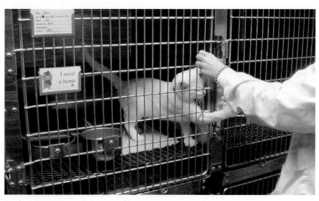

C Once the cat's legs touch the cage floor, let go of its body and regain control of the cage door.

D Quickly let go of the scruff and shut the cage door.

RETURNING TO CAGE OR CARRIER

With the cat on your right hip and your right hand holding the scruff, open the cage door with your left hand (Fig. 3-7, *A*). Use your left hand to support the cat's body while maintaining control of its head with your right hand and lift the cat toward the rear of the cage (Fig. 3-7, *B*).

The cat must be facing away from you. This places its feet and teeth the farthest from your body. Once the cat's legs touch the cage floor, let go of its body and regain control of the cage door (Fig. 3-7, *C*). Quickly let go of the scruff, and shut the cage door (Fig. 3-7, *D*). *Remember to make sure the door is latched tight.*

FIG. 3-8

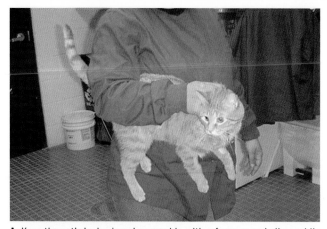

A Keep the cat's body pinned on one hip with a forearm and elbow while retaining control of its head by the scruff.

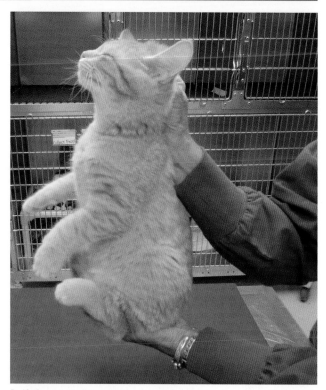

B If the cat really starts to struggle, you can simply release its body from under your arm and hold the cat away from your body by the scruff of its neck.

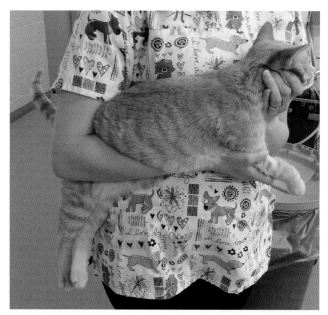

C Wrap the cat across your body, securely holding its head and supporting its body with your forearm and place your fingers between its front legs.

CARRYING A CAT

Keep the cat's body pinned on one hip with a forearm and elbow while retaining control of its head by the scruff (Fig. 3-8, *A*). This frees up your other hand to open and close doors and keeps your free arm away from dangerous front claws and teeth.

If it feels like the cat is slipping, you can adjust the cat higher up on your hip. To do this, place your left hand under the cat's abdomen and shift the cat up. *Caution:* Do not put your free arm (in this case the left arm) around the cat's chest. Cats often feel like the hold is becoming a trap and will struggle more to get free.

If the cat really starts to struggle, you can release its body from under your arm and hold the cat away from your body by the scruff of the neck (Fig. 3-8, *B*). This looks horrible but accomplishes a couple of things. Most cats will settle down and draw their back legs and tail close to their bodies because of the scruffing. This technique also moves the cat's claws away from your body, thus protecting you from serious scratches. Alternately a cat can be carried by using your forearm to support its body, grasping it under the chin, and holding it firmly against your body (Fig. 3-8, *C*).

FIG. 3-9

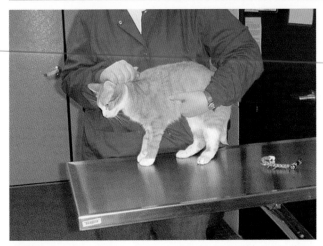

A Maintain control of the head by scruffing the cat with your dominant hand, thumb pointing toward the cat's rear end, and supporting the abdomen with the other.

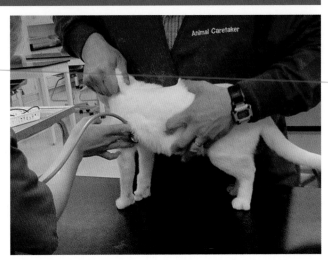

B Present the cat's left side so that the person doing the temperature, pulse, and respiration check has access to the chest for the best auscultation of the heart.

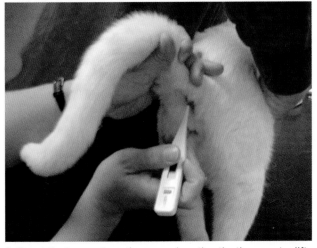

C To get the temperature, the person inserting the thermometer lifts the tail.

RESTRAINT TECHNIQUES

The following are restraint techniques used to perform medical procedures on cats. It takes practice to get good at restraining cats. Cats can feel your confidence, so handling cats gently but firmly will bring you the most success. Students often make the mistake of clamping a cat down in the tightest hold they can get and then are surprised when the cat reacts violently. If you remember to start the hold when the person doing the procedure has everything ready and start with the minimum amount of restraint necessary, you will

be amazed at how well the cat will behave. Be ready to increase your hold or to shift holds quickly if the cat starts to move or resist.

The standing, sternal, and lateral restraint techniques are the basis for almost all other techniques used on cats. They all utilize the head and leg holds previously described in this chapter. Once you master these techniques, you will be able to hold a cat for most procedures, with only slight modifications needed for others.

STANDING RESTRAINT

Maintain control of the head by scruffing the cat with your dominant hand, thumb pointing toward the cat's rear end, and supporting the abdomen with the other (Fig. 3-9, *A*). Keep your elbows tucked close to your body and the cat's body snuggled against yours. This is a good restraint technique for physical examinations. Present the cat's left side so that the person doing the temperature, pulse, and respiration has access to the cat's chest for the best auscultation of the heart (Fig. 3-9, *B*). To get the temperature, the person inserting the thermometer lifts the tail. You, as the restrainer, should be ready for a reaction from the cat, but you should not tighten your hold unless it is necessary. Distraction techniques are appropriate at this time; you can wiggle the cat's body or scruff or blow puffs of air into the cat's face (Fig. 3-9, *C*).

FIG. 3-10

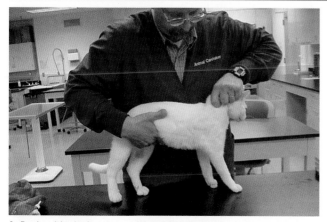

A Begin with placing the cat in standing restraint.

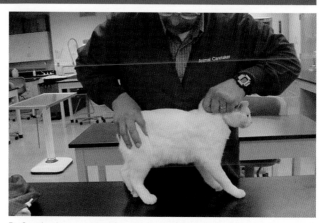

B Gently place your hand on the cat's back near its hips.

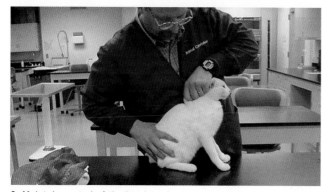

C Maintain control of the head so the cat cannot reach down and bite your hand as it manipulates its front legs.

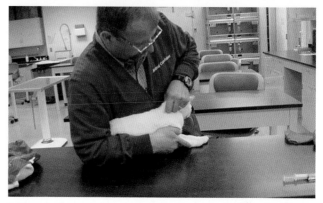

D Use your free arm to snug the cat into your body. Notice that the restrainer's body is slightly over the cat's back.

STERNAL RESTRAINT

Begin by placing the cat in standing restraint (Fig. 3-10, *A*). Gently place your hand on the cat's back near its hips. Push gently to ease the cat into a sitting position (Fig. 3-10, *B*). Once the cat is sitting, gently push down its front legs or pull them down with your free hand. The legs should slide so they rest under the cat's chin. Maintain control of the head so the cat cannot reach down and bite your hand as it manipulates the front legs (Fig. 3-10, *C*). Maintain the cat in sternal position while holding the scruff with a bit of downward pressure. Use your free arm to snug the cat into your body. Notice that your body will be slightly over the cat's back. This maintains the cat in sternal recumbency, but

be careful not to exert too much pressure and squash the cat (Fig. 3-10, *D*)! You can control the cat's front legs by sliding your hand underneath them, palm up, and placing your finger between them as you cradle the cat's elbows in your palm. This prevents the cat from pulling its legs back and scratching the person performing the procedure.

Sternal restraint can be used for many procedures, including the following:

- Cleaning ears (Fig. 3-11, *A*)
- Administering ophthalmic medication (Fig. 3-11, *B*)
- Administering oral liquid medication (Fig. 3-11, *C*)
- Administering oral solid medication (Fig. 3-11, *D*)
- Administering SQ injections (Fig. 3-11, *E*)

FIG. 3-11

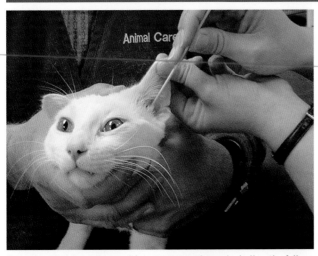

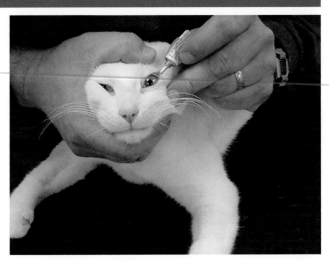

Sternal restraint can be used for many procedures, including the following: **A** Ear cleaning.

B Ophthalmic medication.

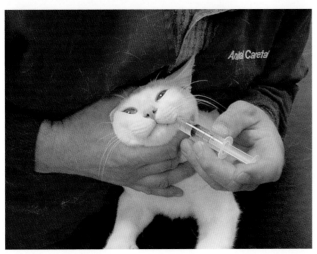

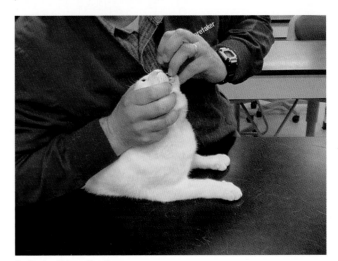

C Oral liquid medication.

D Oral solid medication.

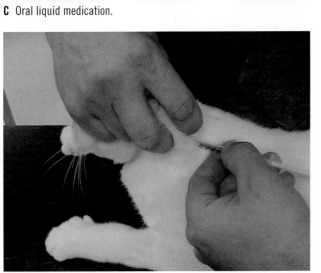

E Subcutaneous injections.

LEFT-LATERAL RECUMBENCY (THE CAT'S LEFT SIDE WILL TOUCH THE TABLE)

With your left hand, scruff the cat with your thumb pointing toward the cat's head. Steady the cat between your arms with the other hand (Fig. 3-12, *A*). Slide your right hand under the cat's back legs, grasping above the hocks and placing your finger between the cat's legs. Maintain control of the cat by keeping your arm right alongside it at all times (Fig. 3-12, *B*). Gently stretch and rotate the cat over on its side onto the table. Lay the cat's back along your forearm.

Stretch the cat the entire length of your forearm. This prevents the cat from using its front legs to scratch and its body from twisting (Fig. 3-12, *C*). Maintain good control of the scruff, and do not let the cat get its left front leg under it or it will be able to stand up. Keep the cat's spine aligned with your arm at all times (Fig. 3-12, *D*). To release the cat, help it regain sternal recumbency by easing the head up and allowing the back legs to move into normal position. Continue to control the head until it is time to return the cat to its cage (Fig. 3-12, *E*).

FIG. 3-12

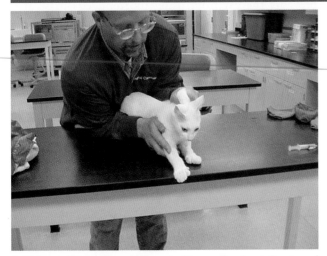

A With your left hand, scruff the cat with your thumb pointing toward the cat's head. Steady the cat between your arms with the other hand.

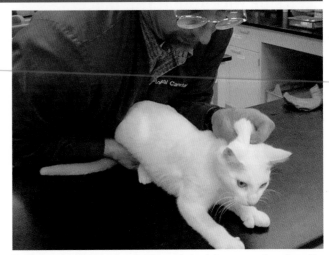

B Slide your right hand under the cat's back legs, grasping above the hocks and placing your finger between the cat's legs.

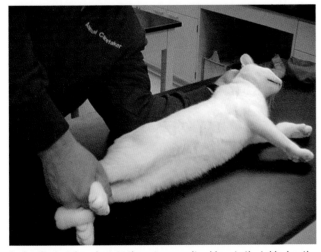

C Gently stretch and rotate the cat over on its side onto the table. Lay the cat's back along your forearm.

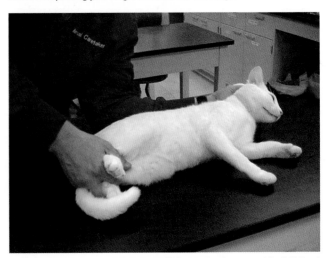

D Maintain good control of the scruff. Do not let the cat get its left front leg under it or the cat will be able to stand up.

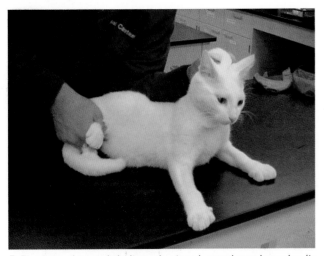

E To release the cat, help it regain sternal recumbency by easing its head up and allowing its back legs to move into normal position.

RIGHT-LATERAL RECUMBENCY (THE CAT'S RIGHT SIDE WILL TOUCH THE TABLE)

This is basically the same technique as left-lateral recumbency. You simply start with your right hand on the scruff and use your left hand to control the cat's back legs (Fig. 3-13). This allows the restrainer to present the other side of the cat for injections or examinations.

TWO-PERSON LATERAL RECUMBENCY

The person giving the injection grasps the cat's back legs with his or her free hand. The restrainer scruffs the cat and holds its front legs with his or her finger in between the legs for added security. Simultaneously both people will stretch the cat so it lies alongside the restrainer's forearm as they lower the cat's body to the table (Fig. 3-14, *A*).

The key to both techniques is to maintain the cat in a full stretch. If allowed to curl up, the cat can twist and get out of the hold fairly easily. Veterinary professionals use lateral recumbency to give both IM and SQ injections, to examine the animal's side, and, if the cat is a bit too naughty, to perform standing restraint during a temperature, pulse, and respiration check (Fig. 3-14, *B*).

FIG. 3-13

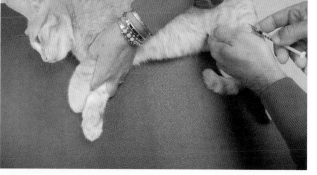

You simply start with the right hand on the scruff and the left hand controlling the back legs.

FIG. 3-14

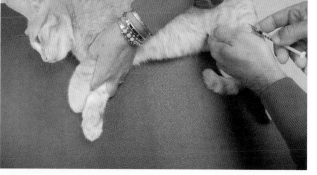

A The restrainer scruffs the cat and holds its front legs with a finger in between the legs for added security.

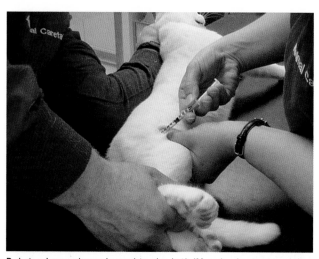

B Lateral recumbency is used to give both IM and subcutaneous injections, to examine the animal's side, and if the cat is a bit naughty for standing restraint during a temperature, pulse, and respiration check.

PRETZEL HOLD

On occasion, a veterinary professional may have to give an IM injection without a helper. One way to accomplish this is by placing the cat into what looks like a pretzel, hence the name. Grasp as much skin as you can over the cat's neck and shoulders. Grasp the back leg (the one that is on the same side as your thumb that is holding the scruff) with the other hand. Bend the cat toward that back leg and quickly hook its hock with your thumb (Fig. 3-15). This presents its *biceps femoris* muscle for an IM injection. Usually the cat will not seem to mind because it is worried about its leg being behind its ears, so if you hurry it will not think to scratch you with its front feet. This hold is not hard on cats if you think about how they clean their back ends! This hold must not be used on obese cats as it may strain a muscle being moved into this position.

FIG. 3-15

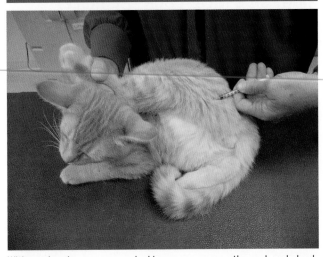

With one hand, grasp as much skin as you can over the neck and shoulders. With your other hand, grasp the back leg that is on the same side as your thumb that is holding the scruff. Bend the cat toward that back leg and quickly hook the hock with your thumb.

RESTRAINT FOR VENIPUNCTURES

Cats often respond negatively to being poked. This often makes the new restrainer nervous, who then holds the cat with a death grip. We've already discussed how the cats respond to being held too tightly and for too long a time. Please do not put the cat into these holds until the person performing the venipuncture has the syringe assembled, cap on the needle loosened, cotton ball soaked, and the collection tube ready to go.

Cephalic venipuncture requires the cat to be in sternal recumbency. Scruff the cat with your right hand, with your thumb pointing toward the cat's back end. Slide the cat to the edge of the table, then bring your left hand around the side of the cat's body and snug it up against your body (Fig. 3-16, *A*). Turn the cat's head away from your partner and toward your body. With your left hand cradling the cat's left elbow, wrap your thumb across the proximal part of the forearm as you extend the left leg forward toward your partner (Fig. 3-16, *B*). Your partner will grasp the cat's foot, which frees your hand to occlude the vessel. To occlude the vessel, keep your thumb in place but roll it laterally so your thumb ends up perpendicular to the vessel. This causes the vessel to stand up and rolls it to the top of the cat's leg for easier access. Continue to hold the cat's elbow securely in the palm of your hand (Fig. 3-16, *C*). For added security, grasp the cat's other leg and pin it between your little finger and palm. This prevents the cat from using it to scratch you or your partner while performing the venipuncture (Fig. 3-16, *D*). Be able to switch hands and hold the scruff with the left hand and the front leg with the right (Fig. 3-16, *E*).

FIG. 3-16

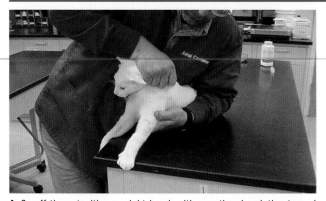

A Scruff the cat with your right hand, with your thumb pointing toward the cat's back end. Slide the cat to the edge of the table and bring your left hand around the side of the cat's body and snug it up against your body.

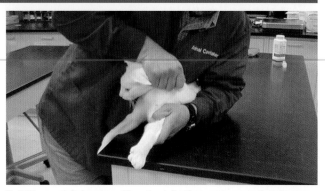

B With your left hand cradling the left elbow, wrap your thumb across the proximal part of the forearm as you extend the left leg forward toward your partner.

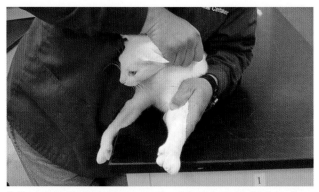

C To occlude the vessel, keep your thumb in place but roll it laterally so your thumb ends up perpendicular to the vessel.

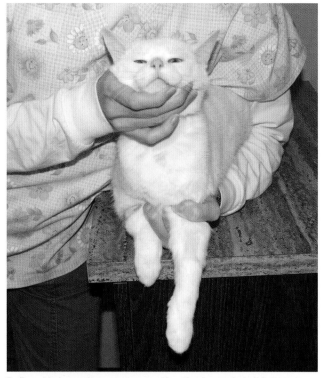

D For added security you can grasp the other leg and pin it between your little finger and palm.

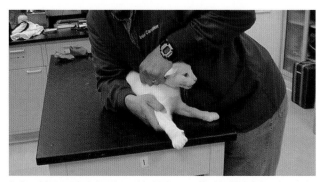

E Be able to switch hands and hold the scruff with the left hand and the front leg with the right.

APPLYING A TOURNIQUET FOR CEPHALIC VENIPUNCTURE

Place the cat in sternal recumbency using the same technique as you would for a cephalic venipuncture. The restrainer extends the limb to be used by cradling the elbow in the palm of the left hand without laying the thumb across the vessel. The phlebotomist slips the tourniquet over the paw (Fig. 3-17, *A*). The tourniquet goes proximal to the elbow and the tails and clip are on the caudolateral aspect of the elbow.

Pull the ends of the tourniquet to tighten. The restrainer reestablishes the hold on the cat's leg so the cat does not pull it back (Fig. 3-17, *B*). To release the tourniquet, grab both sides (top and bottom) of the clip and pull it away from the base as you pull the entire locking mechanism away from the leg (Fig. 3-17, *C*). Use this same technique to place a tourniquet on a dog's limb.

FIG. 3-17

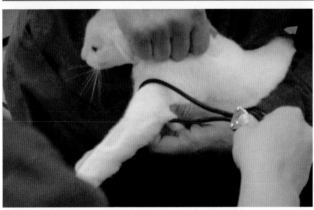

A The restrainer extends the limb to be used by cradling the elbow in the palm of his or her left hand without laying the thumb across the vessel. The phlebotomist slips the tourniquet over the paw.

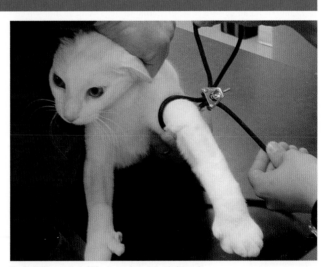

B Pull the ends of the tourniquet to tighten it.

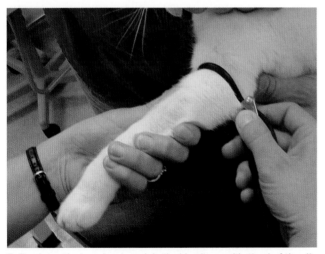

C To release the tourniquet, grab both sides (top and bottom) of the clip and pull it away from the base as you pull the entire locking mechanism away from the leg.

FIG. 3-18

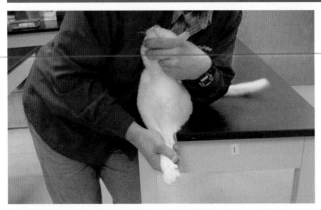

A Extend the head upward while extending the legs down so that you can see the jugular vessel.

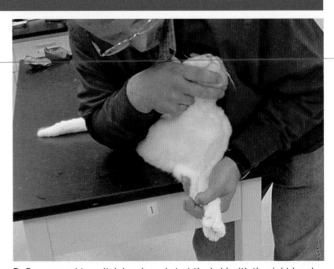

B Be prepared to switch hands and start the hold with the right hand.

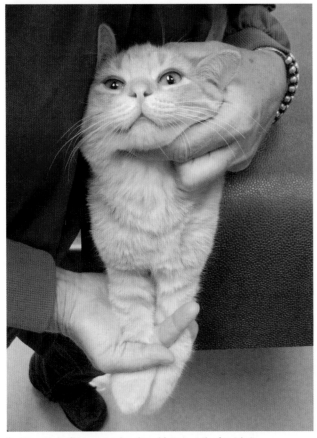

C Alternately, fingers can be placed between the front legs.

There are two holds to use for jugular venipuncture. The first method involves starting just as you would for the cephalic hold. Once to the edge of the table, shift your left hand to a cupping technique with the fingers under the mandible and the thumb on top of the head. Note how the left arm is snugging the cat's body up against the restrainer's chest. Gently move your right hand under the cat and grasp both front legs above the elbows, with your finger in between the legs for added gripping power. Extend the cat's head upward while extending its legs down so that you can see the jugular vessel (Fig. 3-18, *A*). Be prepared to switch hands and start the hold with the right hand (Fig. 3-18, *B*). The difficult part of this hold is getting your fingers out of the way while maintaining control of the cat's head. As you can see in Figure 3-18, *B*, only two fingers are used to hold the head up securely. It takes a lot of practice to develop the strength to hold a cat like this. Placing a finger between the front legs can prevent pain to the cat (Fig. 3-18, *C*). Cats do not tolerate this hold for long. The phlebotomist should have everything ready to go before the restrainer puts the cat into position. This includes wetting the cotton ball, having the needle cover loose, and breaking the seal on the plunger.

The other method is to hold the cat on its back. It is easier to do this if the cat is wrapped in a towel or placed in a cat bag. See the section on equipment for instructions on how to place a cat in a towel or cat bag. Once the cat is wrapped up in the towel, roll it over so it is lying on its back. The restrainer uses one hand to grasp the head from the back and holds the cat's front feet under the towel and down toward its chest. When ready, the phlebotomist takes the cat's head, and the restrainer holds the front feet inside the towel and occludes the vessels. The phlebotomist cups the back of the head in the palm of one hand and lays a thumb across the

FIG. 3-19

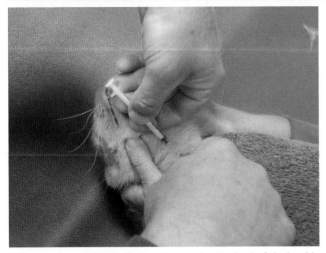

A The phlebotomist holds the head by cupping the back of the head in the palm of her hand and laying her thumb across the mandibles.

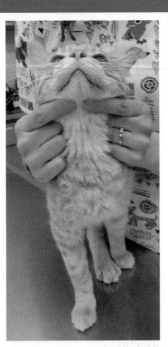

B The restrainer allows the cat to stand while holding each mandible with his or her thumbs under each mandible while his or her fingers are on top of the cat's head.

mandibles (Fig. 3-19, *A*). The phlebotomist has to be careful when holding the head. If the cat should struggle and the phlebotomist's thumb slips down over the trachea, the cat could actually suffocate. Most cats do not object to this hold and seem to stay still a bit longer than they do for the previous technique. An alternative method is to allow the cat to stand while the restrainer places his or her fingers on each side of the head and then lifts, holding under each mandible (Fig. 3-19, *B*). The restrainer must be careful to hold onto the mandibular bone and not occlude the trachea. Many cats respond well to this less restrictive method of restraint.

RESTRAINT FOR NAIL TRIMMING

Place the cat in sternal restraint. Depending on which paw you are treating and which is your dominant hand, one hand will do two tasks. Hold the scruff and the left front paw with the thumb and index fingers of your right hand while your left hand trims the nail. To trim the right front paw, hold it with your little and ring fingers (Fig. 3-20, *A*). To trim the back legs, tuck the cat's head behind your elbow. Do not let go of the scruff until you have control of the cat's head with your elbow (Fig. 3-20, *B*). Hold up one of the cat's back feet and extend the claw with your right hand as you trim with your left. Move to the other foot when you have trimmed all the nails on the first one (Fig. 3-20, *C*). If you are right handed, switch.

RESTRAINT EQUIPMENT

Veterinary professionals can use a number of tools to restrain cats more effectively and safely if they are aggressive or easily agitated.

TOWELS

A large, medium-weight towel works well for restraining most cats for almost every procedure. The towel can be used in a variety of ways.

FIG. 3-20

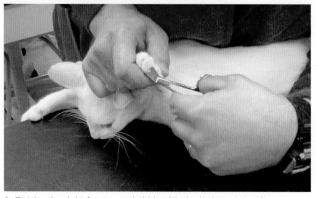

A To trim the right front paw, hold it with the little and ring fingers.

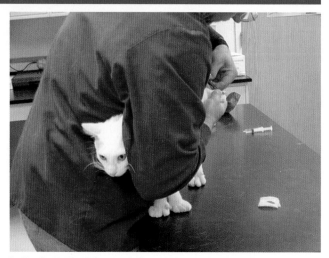

B To trim the back legs tuck the cat's head behind your elbow.

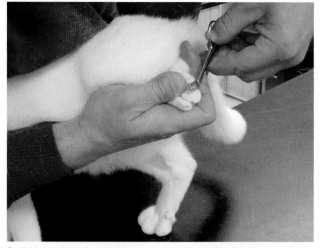

C Hold up a back foot and extend the claw with your right hand and trim with your left.

Start with the towel laid flat on an examination table (Fig. 3-21, *A*). Place the cat in sternal recumbency parallel to the ends of the towel about one third of the way from the end of the towel. Wrap the shortest end tightly around the cat's body, maintaining hold of the scruff (Fig. 3-21, *B*). Continue to wrap the towel tightly around the cat's entire body, much like a burrito, with just the cat's head sticking out (Fig. 3-21, *C*). Once the cat has been wrapped in the towel, check to be sure its neck is snug but its airway is not restricted. The cat should not be able to stand up, even partially, because it can squirm out of the towel if it can get its feet under it.

FIG. 3-21

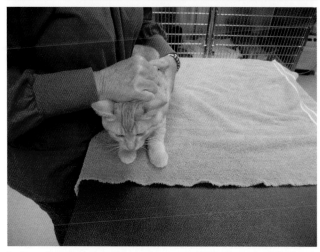

A Place the cat in sternal recumbency parallel to the ends of the towel, about one third of the way from the end of the towel.

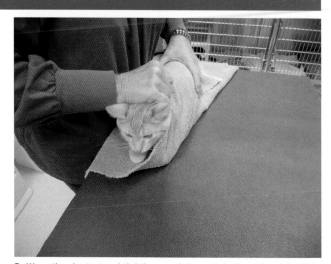

B Wrap the shortest end tightly around the cat's body, maintaining hold of the scruff.

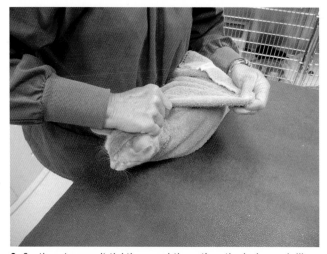

C Continue to wrap it tightly around the cat's entire body, much like a burrito, with just the head sticking out.

(**Figure 3-21**, continued on following page)

FIG. 3-21 cont.

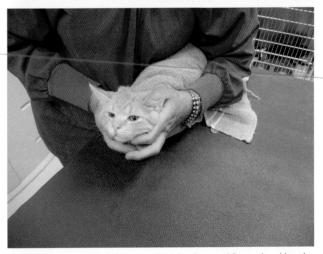

D It also works well for intramuscular injections and femoral and jugular venipunctures by exposing the body part that you require.

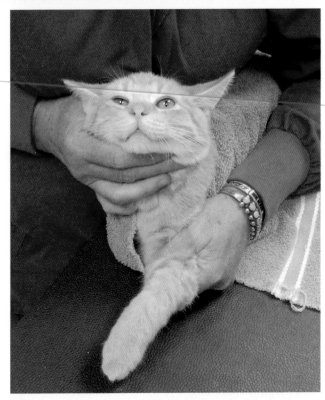

E To remove the cat from the towel, lift the free side of the towel as you lift the cat and unwind the towel.

You can use towel wraps to restrain cats while medicating their eyes or ears and/or to give oral medications when you are all alone or the cat is feisty. Towel wraps also simplify IM injections and femoral and jugular venipunctures by exposing the body part that you are treating (Fig. 3-21, *D*). To remove the cat from the towel, lift the free side of the towel as you lift the cat and unwind the towel. Maintain control of the scruff the entire time (Fig. 3-21, *E*).

BLANKETS

You can throw a blanket that has been folded into quarters or a very thick towel over an aggressive or fearful cat and scoop it up to remove it from a cage or carrier. To do this, fold the thick towel in half and then quickly drop it over the cat with the fold running the length of the cat's body (a lot like a taco with the cat being the filling) (Fig. 3-22, *A*).

With forearms, in gauntlets if you are working with an extremely aggressive cat, reach on either side of the cat's body and sweep its legs out from under it, closing the blanket tightly around the cat as you go. While placing the cat on an examination table, either you can continue to wrap the cat up tight or another person can grasp one of the cat's back legs and give an IM injection (Fig. 3-22, *B*).

FIG. 3-22

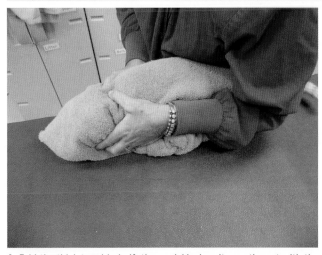
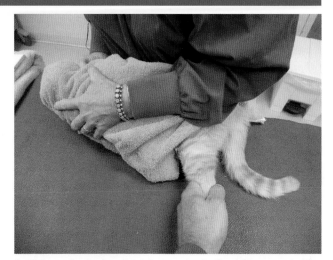

A Fold the thick towel in half, then quickly drop it over the cat with the fold running the length of its body. With forearms, in gauntlets if working with an extremely aggressive cat, reach on either side of the cat's body and sweep the legs out from under it. Close the blanket tightly around the cat as you go.

B While moving to place the cat on an examination table, you can either continue to wrap the cat up tight or another person can grasp a back leg and give an intramuscular injection.

CAT RESTRAINT BAG

The cat restraint bag is a manufactured nylon or canvas bag that is designed to secure a cat's legs and body with a number of strategically placed zippered openings. The key to getting a cat into the bag is speed. Choose the proper-size bag. If the cat bag is too small, you will never get the cat into it; if it is too large, the cat will be able to squirm around. Start by laying the bag open wide on the table, scruff the cat with your right hand, and lift, placing it into sternal recumbency on top of the open bag (Fig. 3-23, *A*). Use your body and scruffing hand to keep the cat down. If it stands up, it will scramble to its feet and bunch the bag up. With your left hand, bring one side of the neck strap up and quickly grasp it with the hand scruffing the cat (Fig. 3-23, *B*). Quickly grasp the other band and bring it under the cat's neck, securely fastening the strap around the neck. Be careful to keep your fingers out of the cat's bite range (Fig. 3-23, *C*). Maintain a downward pressure over the cat's shoulders with your right hand.

Quickly slide your left hand in between the cat's back legs and move them up and toward the thorax, curling the cat's body into the bag. This prevents the cat from standing up and stepping out of the bag (Fig. 3-23, *D*). Bring the sides up and if your bag has a hair guard smooth that into place. Tuck the cat's head tightly between your body and your elbow and zip the bag. Be very careful not to zip the cat's hair, tail, or legs into the zipper (Fig. 3-23, *E*). If your bag does not have a hair guard, grasp the zipper and pull it with your thumb and index finger while sliding your fingers underneath it. As you move your fingers along, push the cat's hair out of the way (Fig. 3-23, *F*). Once you have zipped the bag, quickly gain control of the cat's head (Fig. 3-23, *G*). The cat can still bite. This bag

FIG. 3-23

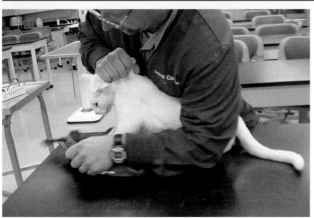

A Start by laying the bag open wide on the table, scruff the cat with your right hand, and lift the cat, placing it into sternal recumbency on top of the open bag.

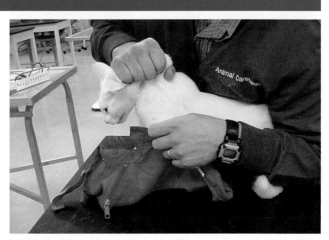

B With the left hand, bring one side of the neck strap up and scruff the cat while holding onto the neck.

(**Figure 3-23,** continued on following page)

FIG. 3-23 cont.

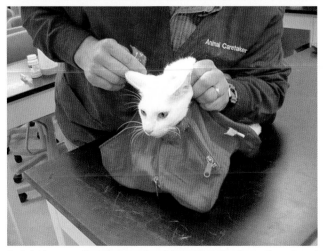

C Quickly grasp the other band and bring it under the cat's neck and securely fasten the bag around the cat's neck.

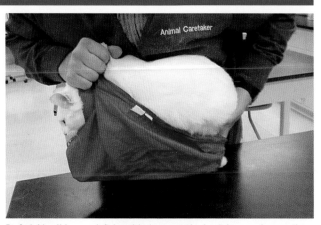

D Quickly slide your left hand in between the back legs and move them up and toward the cat's thorax, curling the cat's body into the bag.

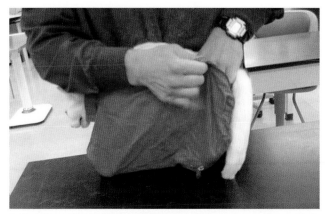

E Tuck the cat's head tightly between your body and your elbow and zip the bag.

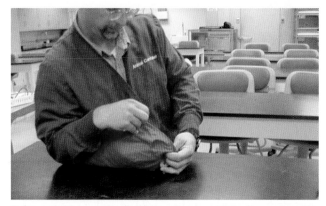

F Grasp the zipper and pull with your thumb and index finger while sliding your fingers underneath the zipper. As you move your fingers along, push the hair out of the way.

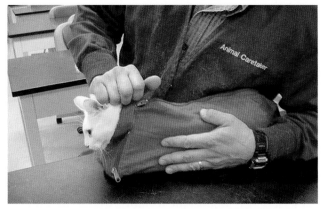

G Once the bag is zipped, quickly gain control of the cat's head.

FIG. 3-24

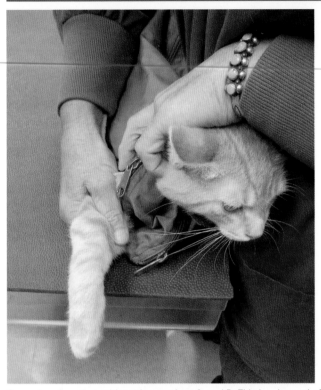
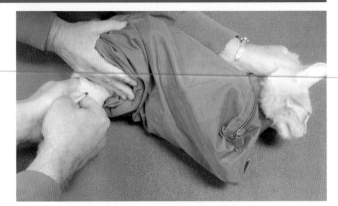

Femoral venipuncture with cat in a cat bag. **A** and **B** This bag is wonderful for cephalic, femoral, and saphenous venipunctures; intramuscular injections; administering medications; and treatments to the head. Note occlusion of the femoral vein by the restrainer.

is wonderful for cephalic, femoral, and saphenous venipunctures, IM injections, administering medications, and treatments to the head (Fig. 3-24, *A* and *B*). *Never leave a cat unattended in a bag!* It can roll off the table and be severely injured.

To remove a cat from a bag, close all of the auxiliary zippers, scruff the cat with your right hand, and unzip the bag with your left. Be very careful not to zip the cat's hair, tail, or legs as you open the zipper. Next, working quickly, release the neck strap and allow the cat to step forward out of the bag. If the cat is wise to the restraint bag, you may need a second person to help you keep the cat's body pushed down until you unzip the bag.

MUZZLES

Many muzzles are of dubious worth on cats. They must be wide enough to cover the cat's entire face, including the eyes, but have an opening that is positioned so that the cat can still breathe through its nose. It is difficult to secure them behind the cat's ears because its head is so rounded and there is not much "ledge" there to keep the strap from moving forward. The restrainer may inadvertently pull the muzzle off if the cat moves its head or body violently.

If using nylon muzzles, choose the proper-size muzzle. Be sure you know which side goes up. Cats usually only give you one chance to get the muzzle in place. Place the cat in sternal recumbency. Hold one tab of the muzzle in your hand as you scruff the cat with your thumb pointing toward the cat's head. Use your forearm to snug the cat close to your body (Fig. 3-25, *A*). With your other hand, grasp the very end of the other tab and swing wide to avoid the mouth, then bring the muzzle over the cat's face (Fig. 3-25, *B*). Secure the muzzle tabs behind the ears as low and tight as they will go (Fig. 3-25, *C* and *D*).

Check that the muzzle does not cover the cat's nares. If they are covered, the cat will panic because it cannot breathe and will struggle to be free of the muzzle.

To remove the muzzle, scruff the cat and quickly release the tabs and pull the muzzle away from the cat's face. It is important to move your hand quickly away from the cat's mouth so that the cat does not bite you.

Solid-cone–type muzzles can also be used and tend to be a bit easier to place. They are slipped over the entire head and tied behind the ears (Fig. 3-25, *E* and *F*).

FIG. 3-25

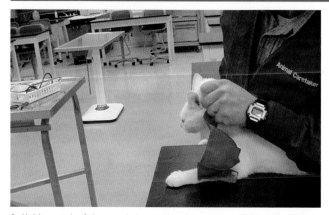
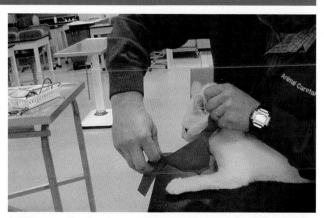

A Hold one tab of the muzzle in your hand as you scruff the cat with your thumb pointing toward the cat's head. Snug the cat to your body by using your forearm to slide it close.

B With your other hand, grasp the very end of the other tab and swing wide to avoid the mouth, then bring the muzzle over the cat's face.

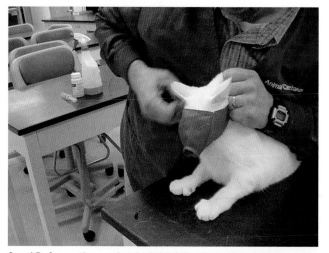
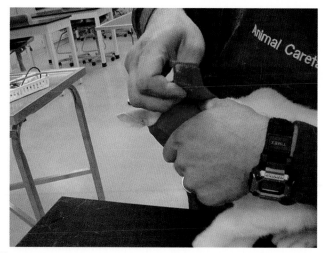

C and D Secure the muzzle tabs behind the ears as low and tight as they will go.

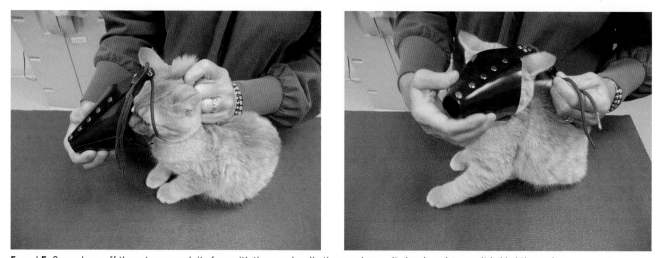

E and **F** Securely scruff the cat, approach its face with the muzzle, slip the muzzle over its head, and secure it behind the neck.

FIG. 3-26

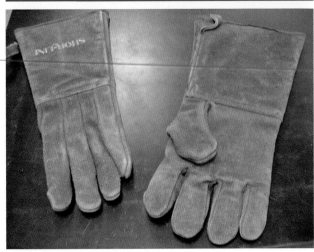

Gauntlets are heavy leather gloves that reach up to the elbow.

GAUNTLETS

These are heavy leather gloves that reach up to the elbow (Fig. 3-26). Use them to protect yourself when the cat is obviously aggressive. Cats can bite through a glove, but it does slow them down enough so that you can move your hand out of the glove before the cat has a chance to penetrate. Gauntlets deflect scratches very well. Take care when holding onto the cat with the gauntlets on, as they do reduce your tactile feeling and you may be gripping the cat harder than you realize. The best way to use gauntlets is as a distraction technique. Place one hand halfway in one glove, put the other hand all the way in the other glove, reach into the cage or carrier with the "dummy" glove, and while the cat is batting at or biting that empty glove, reach around with the other hand and scruff the cat. Lift the cat out of the cage and place it on the examination table.

CHEMICAL RESTRAINT

An inhalation chamber is a great tool that can be used for cats that will not surrender no matter what you do. You can place them in the chamber and use isoflurane or sevoflurane to anesthetize them. The only drawback to using this technique is that the animals do not stay asleep for very long, so you either have to work fast or you must insert an endotracheal tube and keep them on the inhalant gas until your procedure is completed.

FIG. 3-27

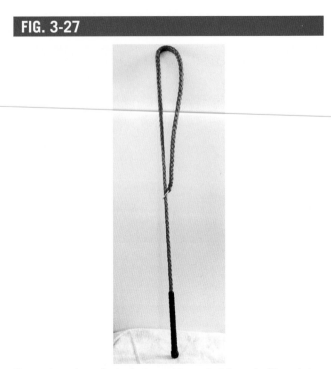

The cat lasso is really the last resort for restraining cats. The pole has a noose at one end that draws tight when placed around the cat's body.

Another chemical restraint technique is to squirt ketamine into the mouth. It is absorbed by the mucous membranes, and the cat is sedated. It is easier to do this than it sounds. Load a dose of ketamine into a syringe with a tomcat catheter attached to the tip and, as the cat hisses, fire away. You may have to fire a couple of times to get the entire dose into the cat, but it works like a charm. This is much easier than trying to give the cat a sedative by an IM injection.

CAT LASSO

The cat lasso is really a tool of last resort to use on cats (Fig. 3-27). The pole has a noose at one end that draws tight when placed around the cat's body. If the noose can be placed around the cat's shoulders, you avoid choking it. If you capture it around the neck, the cat will often react violently because it feels threatened by this hold. If the cat is so wild that you have to use the cat lasso, it is best to put the cat directly into the inhalation chamber or quickly give it a sedative.

SUGGESTED READINGS

Fowler ME: *Restraint and handling of wild and domestic animals*, Ames, IA, 1978, Iowa State University Press, pp 148–155.

Gilbert SG: *Pictorial anatomy of the cat*, New York, 1984, Crescent Books.

Kay D: Fraternizing with fractious felines, *Vet Tech* 5:190–191, 1984.

Kazmierczak K: Bandage management in small animals, *Vet Tech* 3:309–315, 1982.

Leahy JR, Barrow P: *Restraint of animals*, Ithaca, NY, 1953, Cornell Campus Store, pp 164–180.

Medication and force feeding a cat at home, *Client information series*, Schaumburg, IL, 1985, AVMA.

Moran HC, et al: Basic cat handling techniques, *Lab Anim* 29–34, March 1988.

Sayer A: *The complete book of the cat*, New York, 1984, Crescent Books.

Sonsthagen TF: *Restraint of domestic animals*, St. Louis, 1991, Mosby.

Todd-Jenkins K, Dugan B, Remsburg DW, Montgomery C: Restraint and handling of animals. In *McCurnin's clinical textbook for veterinary technicians*, ed 8, Philadelphia, 2014, Saunders.

4

Restraint of Dogs

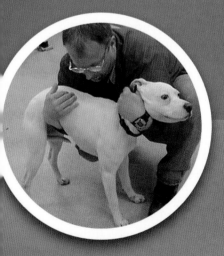
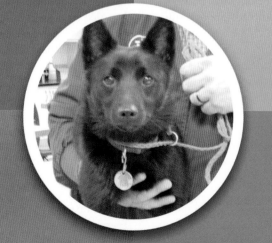
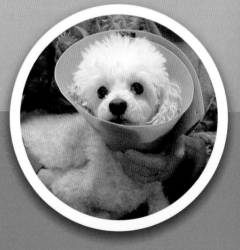

GENERAL CONSIDERATIONS

Most dogs brought to veterinary facilities are friendly and require minimal restraint. However, it is best to be cautious with every dog. All animals can become startled or anxious in a medical facility. The proper way to approach an unknown dog is to extend your hand palm down, with fingers bent slightly toward your palm, allowing the dog to sniff the back of your hand. Watch the dog's reaction and avoid direct eye contact. A friendly dog's body will be relaxed, and the animal will actively sniff your hand, wag its tail, and eventually lose interest in the offered hand. You can then begin gently scratching below the dog's ear, advancing to its chest, neck, shoulders, and top of its hips. A friendly dog at this point trusts you enough to allow restraint holds.

Even friendly dogs must be disciplined on occasion. When you need to discipline a dog, keep in mind that dogs have retained some of the pack instincts of their wild ancestors. In wolf packs, for example, the alpha wolf (male or female), or leader of the pack, keeps order by dominance over the other animals. The domestic bitch instills these same traits in her puppies in much the same way as the alpha wolf does. It will use icy stares, low growls, direct eye contact, and, if necessary, shakes and swats. We can often control unruly patients by imitating the pack leader's dominant behavior.

For example, if you must reprimand a patient, start by looking the dog in the eye and firmly saying, "Spot, enough!" Use a low, stern tone and draw out any "f" or "r" sounds, such as "grrrrrruff" (sounds like low growls).

If the dog does not settle down, you may have to use a physical reprimand. One technique is to grasp the dog's skin on the sides of its neck just behind its jaw. Elevate its head so you can look it in the eye and give it a quick shake, again repeating, *"Enough!"* Do not maintain this hold or eye-to-eye contact for longer than a few seconds. If it is not immediately successful, the dog may be aggressive and accept the "challenge" of a direct stare by coming at you. Another method is to gently "chuck" the dog under the chin with the open hand and repeat the "Enough!"

For any reprimand to be effective, it must be given immediately after the offense has occurred. If you do not strictly observe this timing, the dog may not respond to your reprimand.

It is generally advisable not to physically reprimand a dog in front of its owner, as that can be misinterpreted as cruelty. If the dog is being unruly in the client's presence, it is best to politely ask the client to wait in the reception area or move the dog into another area of the hospital. When separated from their owners, most dogs calm down and are easier to work with because they are not protecting their owners. Also, the client is not there to undermine any dominance you might have gained over the dog.

A cardinal rule is to never have a client restrain his or her own animal. This is important for several reasons. First, clients usually do not know the restraint techniques necessary for various procedures. The second and more important reason is that the veterinarian is liable if the owner is bitten.

If the dog has behaved well during restraint, liberally praise it in clipped, constructive tonalities. Use a normal-sounding but excited voice to say, "Good dog! Well done!" Do not use a high-pitched, squeaky voice that the dog may associate with littermate sounds. This can cause the dog to think of you as an equal, which reduces your social standing in its eyes. Try not to go overboard with the praise; it should be short and sweet. It should also be given the instant the dog is doing what you wish as this indicates to the dog what you want it to do.

A trip to the veterinary clinic is, for many dogs, a traumatic experience. The different smells and the close proximity of other dogs can cause anxiety in even the best-behaved pet. Fortunately, most dogs respond to being petted and spoken to while any type of procedure is being done. A low soft voice, gentle strokes, slow deliberate movements, and a genuine concern for the dog not only relieve the dog's fears, but also impress the dog's owner.

POTENTIAL FOR INJURY

A dog's canine teeth can be very formidable weapons. Always approach an unfamiliar dog with the idea that it will bite if given the chance. Some breeds are notorious biters, such as chihuahuas, pomeranians, poodles, cocker spaniels, rottweilers, and German shepherds. Not all individual dogs of these breeds are biters, but such reputations are usually well earned.

SPECIAL HANDLING

It would be wonderful if all dogs could be treated and handled the same way. However, considerations must be given to their size, shape, condition, and personality. Puppies, pregnant bitches, and old animals, as well as nervous, aggressive, and injured dogs, all require special handling, not only for the safety of the animal but also for the safety of the handler.

Puppies

Puppies are full of energy and must be watched constantly. Never place them on examination tables or countertops without making sure that your hand is always in contact with them, as they are likely to fall and injure themselves.

When procedures are performed on puppies of any breed, most sit calmly and offer no resistance. If they do squirm or try to get free, lift them up and snug them close to your body. Remember to use your "mommy" dog voice when they are being naughty and your calm and friendly voice when they are being good.

Pregnant Bitches

In the advanced stages of pregnancy, applying excessive pressure on the dog's abdominal organs during restraint can have severe repercussions. When restraining a pregnant bitch, always be aware of where your hands are and how much pressure you are applying to the dog's abdomen.

Old Dogs

Old dogs often are pampered pets accustomed to being treated gently. Their joints can be arthritic and should not be maneuvered into awkward positions. Gentle handling is the key to working with the "old-timers."

Nervous Dogs

Nervous dogs must be handled with great caution, as they can be easily provoked to bite. You can recognize a nervous dog by its shivering, anxious expression, cowering, rapid head and ear movements, and ducking of its head.

These animals often try to flee from situations; if a dog is cornered, never grab at it as it goes by because its instinctive reaction is to bite at the hand preventing it from reaching freedom. You might calm some of these "fear biters" by moving slowly, kneeling down to the dog's level, and softly talking it out of its fears. Offer your hand for sniffing. If the dog pulls its lips back in a grimace or growls, it is best to retreat and handle it as an aggressive dog.

Aggressive Dogs

Occasionally animals do not accept your friendly advances and warn you off with a growl or some other form of body language. Signs of aggression, however, may be difficult to perceive. Some dogs bite with little or no warning. Signs of impending aggression include a head held low, either below or level with the dog's shoulders; direct eye contact; raised hair along the back, ears down, and tail straight out; and an ominous growl or snarl. Dogs showing any of these signs should be handled with extreme caution and must always be considered dangerous.

When you must handle an aggressive dog, two or more people should be involved. If one person gets into trouble, the other can help or bring help. Some handlers do not look directly at an aggressive dog and stand sideways instead of facing the dog straight on. Both of these signals are considered nonchallenging in canine body language. Aggressive dogs may answer a challenge if you inadvertently exhibit challenging body language. If you are attacked by a dog, you should try to escape into another room; if that is not possible, remain still, curl into a fetal position if pulled down or hold on firmly to a solid object if standing, protect your face and throat, and scream for help.

Injured Dogs

Injured dogs must always be treated with extreme caution and care. As a rule, an injured dog should be muzzled before being moved or handled. The exception to this rule is if the dog has an injury to the head or is vomiting. Care must be taken not to jar or twist broken bones when transporting these animals. The best way to transport an injured animal is on a stretcher or flat board. If neither of these is available, a towel or blanket can work well, depending on the animal's size.

To use a blanket or towel for transportation, move the animal onto the blanket by supporting all portions of its body. Two or more people may be required to lift and shift the body. Once the animal is on the blanket, you can move it by lifting up on the corner of the blanket. Be careful to keep the blanket as level as possible so the animal does not roll off.

HANDLING CAGED DOGS

Most dogs welcome the opportunity to leave their cage and meet you at the door with tail wagging. Your main concern is to keep them from jumping to the floor and possibly injuring themselves.

The first step in removing a dog from a cage is to greet the animal. Call the dog's name to get its attention. Never reach into the cage and touch the dog if it is sleeping. This could startle the dog and it may bite.

To remove a small dog (less than 35 lbs) from a cage, call it to the front of the cage and slip your arm around the dog's head, then pull its trunk toward you while maintaining head control (Fig. 4-1, *A*). Place one hand between the dog's front legs and gently slide the dog over so that its body is facing the same way as you are. Use your elbow to clamp its rear quarters against your side. With your free hand, apply a loose "manual" muzzle, with your thumb over the bridge of the dog's nose and your fingers wrapped around its mandible (Fig. 4-1, *B*). Lift the dog clear of the cage to transport it. If you must carry the dog any distance, it is often easier to carry it with your arms wrapped around all four legs and its body held against your chest. Be sure to maintain head control (Fig. 4-1, *C*). This method allows the dog's head to be free, so use a muzzle if you expect the dog to bite.

FIG. 4-1

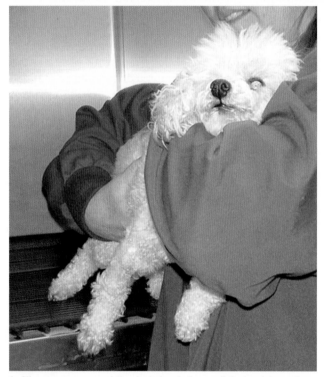

A Slip your arm around the dog's head, then pull its trunk toward you while maintaining head control.

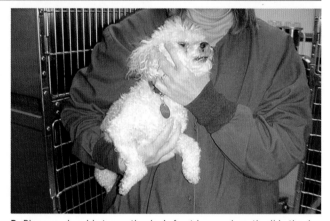

B Place one hand between the dog's front legs and gently slide the dog over so that its body is facing the same way you are. Use your elbow to clamp its rear quarters against your side. With your free hand, apply a loose "manual" muzzle, with your thumb over the bridge of the dog's nose and your fingers wrapped around the mandible.

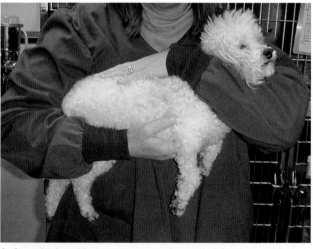

C Carry the dog with your arms wrapped around all four legs and its body held against your chest. Be sure to maintain head control.

LARGE FRIENDLY OR CALM DOGS

Large dogs (more than 35 lbs) generally are kept in large cages at floor level, or they may be housed in runs. A friendly dog is relatively easy to remove. Greet the dog by name or call out to it to be sure it is not sleeping. Open a loop on the rope leash twice the size of the dog's head (Fig. 4-2, *A*). Assess the dog's behavior. If the dog is unfriendly, open the door a small crack, using it as a primary barrier. This barrier keeps the dog in the cage until you can get a leash over its head. If the dog is friendly, you can open the door wider, but continue to use the door as a barrier to prevent the dog from escaping (Fig. 4-2, *B*). Place your leg in front of the cage door to maintain control of the door so that the dog does not barge out. Working through the opening in the cage door, place the loop over the top of the dog's head. Lower the loop and slip it around the dog's neck (Fig. 4-2, *C*). Tighten the leash so it is snug around the dog's neck. Then maintain control of the head by pulling up on the leash. Keep the door closed until you have control of the dog's head (Fig. 4-2, *D*). Open the door and allow the dog to step out while maintaining a tight leash, which will control the dog's head. Quickly remove the dog from the kennel area to prevent provoking nearby animals. It is beneficial to talk to the dog to reassure it.

FIG. 4-2

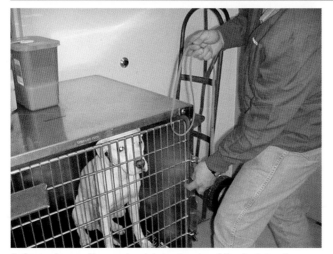

A   Open a loop on the rope leash twice the size of the dog's head.

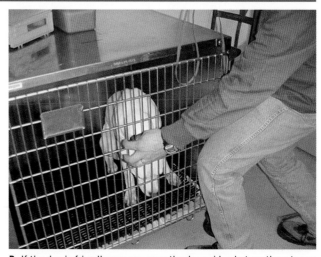

B   If the dog is friendly, you can open the door wider, but continue to use the door as a barrier to prevent the dog from escaping.

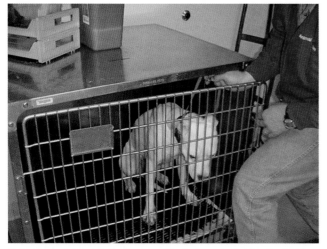

C   Lower the loop and slip it around the dog's neck. Tighten the leash so it is snug around the dog's neck.

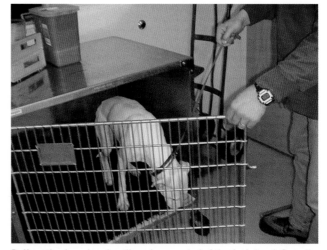

D   Keep the door closed until you have control of the dog's head. Open the door and allow the dog to step out while maintaining a tight leash, which will control the dog's head.

To return a dog to its cage, open and hold the cage door with your left hand (Fig. 4-3, *A*). Hold onto the leash with the other hand, keeping the leash tight to control the dog's head. Ask the dog to "kennel up" and pull on the leash to indicate the direction of travel. If the dog walks into the cage, gently turn the dog so its head is pointed toward the door. Maintain control of the door and the dog's head. If the dog does not walk in, let go of the door and boost the dog into the kennel by reaching between its back legs and lifting up while pushing forward. Maintain control of the head with the leash so the dog cannot swing around and bite you (Fig. 4-3, *B*). To form a barrier so the dog cannot barge through, place your leg in front of the cage door. Thread the handle end of the leash through the cage door or over the top of the door. Reach through the space at the top of the door and pull the loop from around the dog's neck (Fig. 4-3, *C*). Double-check that the cage door is fastened completely. Record what was done to the animal in its medical record (Fig. 4-3, *D*).

Note that it is usually best not to use chain leashes because they can severely injure your hand if the dog attempts to run or begins to struggle violently.

FIG. 4-3

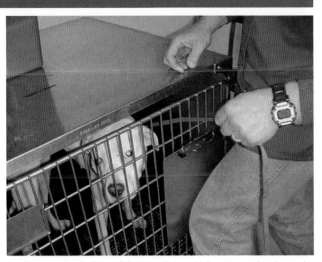

A Open and hold the cage door with your left hand.

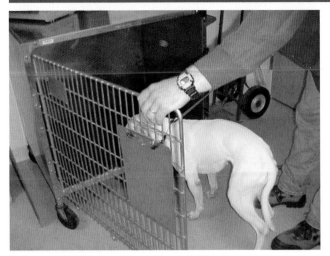

B Place your leg in front of the cage door, which acts as a barrier so the dog cannot barge through.

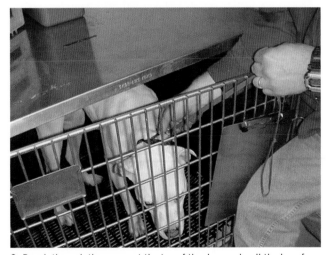

C Reach through the space at the top of the door and pull the loop from around the dog's neck.

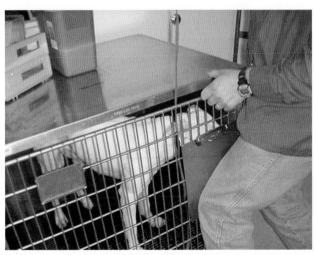

D Double check that the cage door is fastened completely.

NERVOUS OR AGGRESSIVE DOGS

Occasionally a frightened or nervous dog will not allow you to touch it or the cage. In these situations it is best to try to lure the animal out of the cage with quiet, gentle urgings, standing clear of the door and allowing it to walk out on its own. Of course, do this only when the dog is in a ground-level cage. Allowing the dog out of its territory and into strange surroundings often calms it down. Slowly approach the dog and slip the loop of the leash around its head. Before you allow the dog out of the cage, be sure all avenues of escape have been sealed off. Once out of the cage, the dog may try to flee. Remember not to grab at the animal with your bare hands because its natural reaction is to turn and bite.

If the dog is aggressive and you need it out of the cage, use a capture pole (Fig. 4-4, *A*). Open the door wide enough to run the capture pole through it. Make the loop large enough to slip around the dog's head, pulling it tight as it passes the ears (Fig. 4-4, *B*). Some dogs twist and struggle fiercely once they are captured. Hold the dog away from your body and the loop tight. It could be very bad if the dog escaped from the capture pole at this time. You can now lead the dog out of the run and sedate it (Fig. 4-4, *C*).

If you have used a rope leash, as described earlier, you can restrain a struggling dog by running the leash through the cage bars and snubbing its head against the door (Fig. 4-4, *D*). When the dog is subdued, you can call for help and cross-tie the dog, i.e., apply another leash around the neck so that both you and your helper can maintain a tight hold on the head by keeping the leashes tight (Fig. 4-4, *E*). You can give the dog a sedative in the back leg without fear of the dog turning its head as long as the people on the leashes keep them tight.

FIG. 4-4

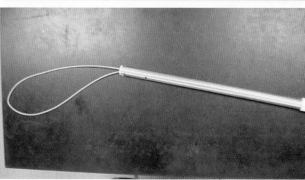

A If the dog is aggressive and you need it out of the cage, use a capture pole.

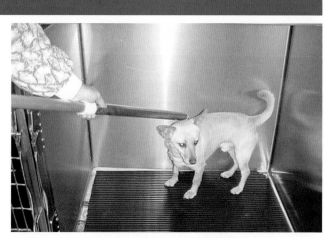

B Slip the loop around the dog's head and pull it tight.

(**Figure 4-4,** continued on following page)

FIG. 4-4 cont.

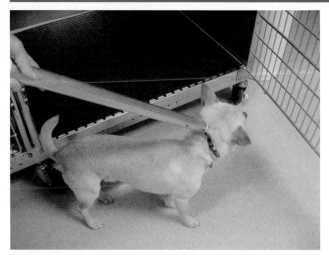

C You can now lead the dog can out of the run and sedate it.

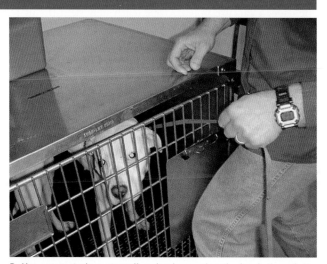

D You can restrain a struggling dog by running the leash through the cage bars and snubbing the dog's head against the door.

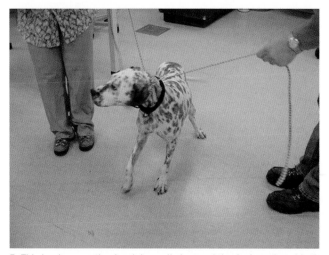

E This is where another leash is applied around the dog's neck and both people maintain a tight hold on the dog's head by keeping the leashes tight.

For smaller dogs that refuse to move from the back of the cage, a capture pole or rope leash may be difficult to maneuver. You can use a large towel or blanket to cover the animal and quickly pick it up and out of the cage. Or you can use gauntlets to grasp the animal. Take one leather glove and place it only partially on your nondominant hand. *Do not* place your fingers all the way into the glove (Fig. 4-5, *A*). Present this partially gloved hand to the dog. While it attacks that near-empty glove, use your other, fully gloved, hand to grasp the dog by the scruff of the neck (Fig. 4-5, *B*). Continue to distract the dog with the empty glove until you can get it to an examination table and muzzle it.

HANDLING DOGS IN A RUN

RETRIEVAL FROM A RUN

To retrieve a dog from a run, call out to the dog to get its attention. Determine its behavior and temperament. If friendly, proceed with getting it out of the run. If unfriendly, go to the section Nervous or Aggressive Dogs. Determine how the latch works and which direction the door swings open (Fig. 4-6, *A*). For a door that opens right to left, unlatch the door and open it just a crack with your

FIG. 4-5

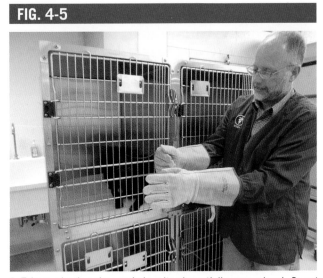

A Take one leather glove and place it only partially on your hand. *Do not* place your fingers all the way into the glove.

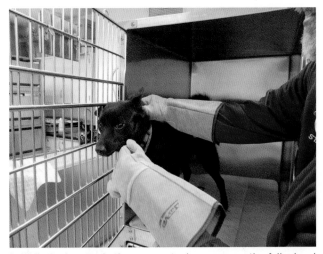

B While the dog attacks the near-empty glove, use your other fully gloved hand to grasp the dog by the scruff of its neck.

FIG. 4-6

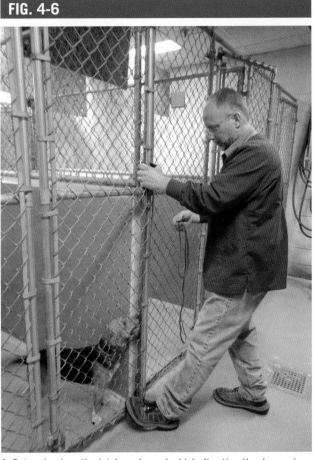

A Determine how the latch works and which direction the door swings open.

(**Figure 4-6,** continued on following page)

left hand while your left leg blocks the door so that the dog cannot push past you (Fig. 4-6, *B*). Form a loop in the rope leash and hold it open with your right hand. Open the door wide enough to slip your arm through and maneuver the leash around the dog's neck. Quickly slip the leash over the dog's neck and tighten the leash. Maintain tension on the leash so that you have control of the dog's

head. If the dog ducks or turns its head, wiggle the door or talk to the dog as a distraction. Keep the run door blocked with your leg until the leash is firmly around the dog's neck (Fig. 4-6, *C*). Once the dog's head has been caught in the leash, you can open the run and allow the dog to walk out of the run. Close the run door. Quickly move the dog out of the run area to avoid provoking other dogs.

FIG. 4-6 cont.

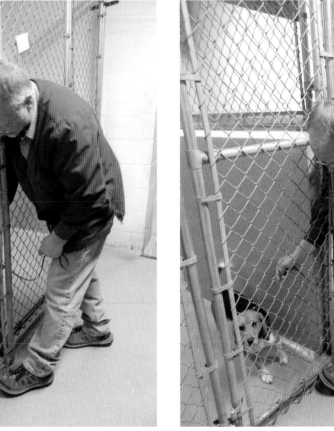

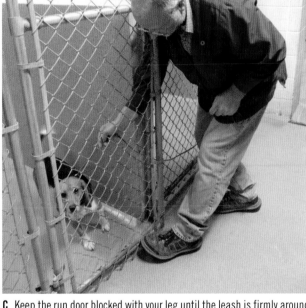

B Unlatch the door and open it just a crack with your left hand while your left leg blocks the door so that the dog cannot push past you.

C Keep the run door blocked with your leg until the leash is firmly around the dog's neck.

RETURNING TO THE RUN

To return a dog to the run, quickly move to the appropriate run and open the door (Fig. 4-7, *A*). Allow the dog to walk in with the command "kennel up." If the dog will not go in, steer it into the run with the leash turning it so its head points toward the door. Once the dog has entered the run, close the door just enough so you can get your arm in and block the door with your leg (Fig. 4-7, *B*). (Figure note: To allow you to see the dog, the restrainer's body is not turned to block the door. Normally, the restrainer's body should be blocking the door.) Reach in and thread the leash through the run door while maintaining head control (Fig. 4-7, *C*). Tip the dog's head away from you by pulling on the leash. Grasp the leash at the back of the animal's neck while your other hand holds the leash tight. Pull the leash off the dog's head and through the door. Securely latch the door. Remember, some dogs will bite or attack you if you simply walk into the run when returning the dog; never turn your back on a dog and walk out.

FIG. 4-7

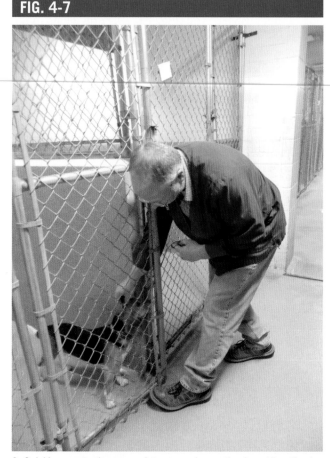

A Quickly move to the appropriate run and open the door. Allow the dog to walk in with the command "kennel up."

(**Figure 4-7,** continued on following page)

FIG. 4-7 cont.

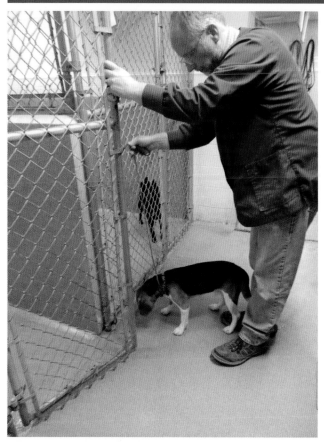

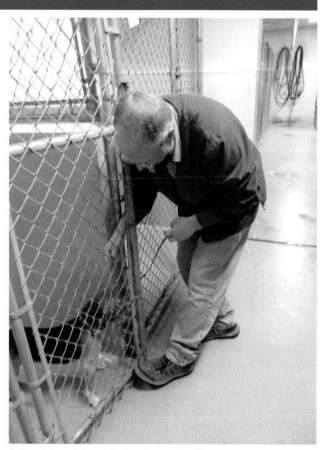

B Once the dog has entered the run, close the door just enough so you can get your arm in and block the door with your leg.

C Reach in and thread the leash through the run door while maintaining head control.

LIFTING AND CARRYING DOGS

Before you lift any dog, consider your safety and the safety of the animal. Always talk to the dog and approach it from the side, not from the front. Remember that approaching a dog from the front may constitute a challenging gesture. If the dog begins to struggle as you are picking it up, hug it closer to your chest, or set it down and start over with more comforting talk. To avoid injuring your back, always squat down and lift with your legs. **Do not** bend over to lift with your back. Keep the weight of the dog evenly distributed to help protect your back from strain.

Lifting and carrying small dogs were discussed in the section on handling caged dogs. One person should be able to lift and carry a 5- to 50-lb dog; a larger dog may require two people to lift and carry it.

LIFTING AND CARRYING A 5- TO 50-POUND DOG

To lift and carry a dog up to 50 lbs, maintain control of the dog's head with the leash. Start this procedure by placing the leash in your right hand. This controls the head by turning it away from you (Fig. 4-8, *A*). Sweep your left hand and arm under and around the neck to gain control of the dog's head. Once you gain head control with your left arm, gather the leash with your right hand and pass it to the left. Slip your right arm under the dog's abdomen, close to its rear legs, and slide the dog close to your body. With knees bent so that you lift with your legs and not your back, lift the dog up. Hold the dog close to your body and talk to it to keep it calm (Fig. 4-8, *B*). Move to the examination table and set the dog down. *Be sure to maintain control of the head* (Fig. 4-8, *C*)! Once the animal is settled, bring the right arm from under the abdomen and remove the leash. Then return to holding the abdomen with the right arm (Fig. 4-8, *D*). Put the leash in your pocket so you have it available when you complete the procedure (Fig. 4-8, *E* and *F*).

FIG. 4-8

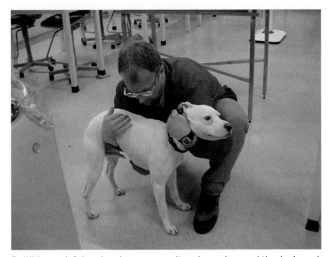

A Maintain control of the dog's head with the leash. Start this procedure by placing the leash in your right hand.

B With your left hand and arm, sweep it under and around the dog's neck to gain control of its head. Slip the right arm under the dog's abdomen, close to its rear legs, and slide the dog close to your body.

(**Figure 4-8,** continued on following page)

FIG. 4-8 cont.

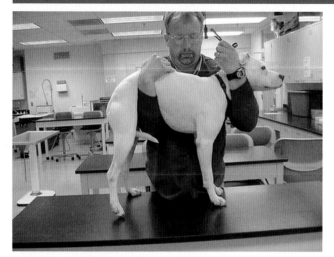

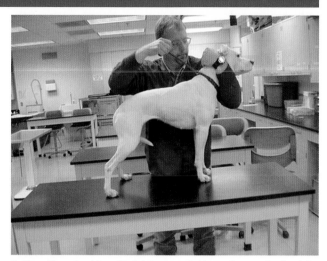

C Slip your right arm under the dog's abdomen, close to its rear legs, and slide the dog close to your body.

D Once the animal is settled, bring your right arm from under its abdomen and remove the leash.

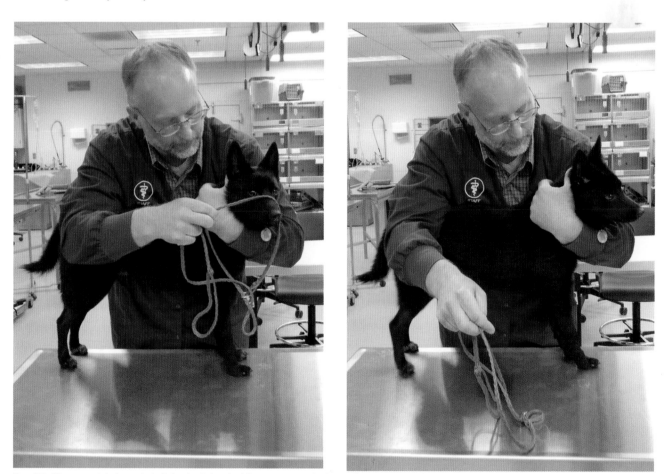

E and **F** Always maintain control of the dog's head while you remove the leash. Be sure not to place your hand in front of the dog's muzzle.

To take the dog off the table, make sure that the dog is in proper standing restraint and briefly let go with the right arm so that you can slip the leash around the animal's neck with your right hand. This allows you to get the leash on without letting go of the dog's head (Fig. 4-9, *A*). Gather the leash with your left hand, again without letting go of the dog's head. Slide the dog close to your body and lift it up and away from the table (Fig. 4-9, *B*). Maintain good head control with one arm while the other supports the animal's abdomen as you lower the dog to the ground. Remember to bend with your knees and not your back (Fig. 4-9, *C*). Once the animal's feet touch the ground, grasp the leash with your right hand while you maintain control of the dog's head with your left arm, which is still around its neck (Fig. 4-9, *D*). As you stand up, remove your left arm and extend your right arm to tighten the leash. The animal is ready to be led off to its owner or returned to the cage.

FIG. 4-9

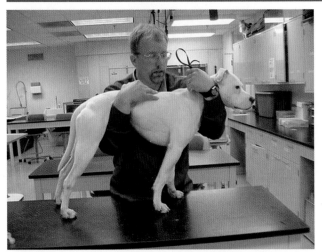

A With the dog in proper standing restraint, briefly let go with the right arm so that you can slip the leash around the animal's neck with your right hand.

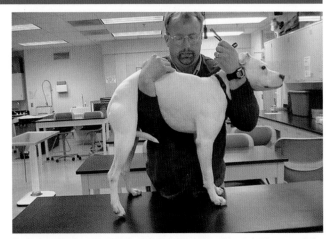

B Gather the leash with the left hand again without letting go of the dog's head. Slide the dog close to your body and lift it up and away from the table.

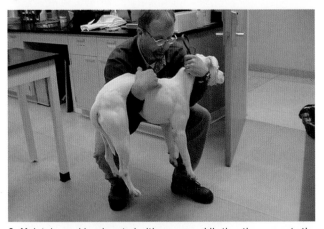

C Maintain good head control with one arm while the other supports the animal's abdomen as you lower the dog to the ground.

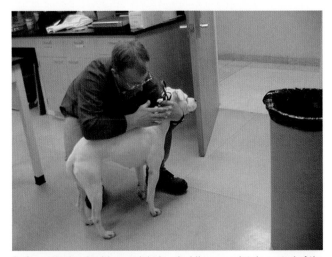

D Grasp the leash with your right hand while you maintain control of the animal's head with your left arm, which is still around the dog's neck.

Carry puppies and small dogs by resting the dog's chest on your forearm, with your fingers between their front legs for a surer grip. Use the other hand to support the dog's head under the chin or place it on top of the dog's neck to minimize wiggling (Fig. 4-10). A word of caution: when the examination is over, never allow the dog to jump from the examination table. Most clinics have stainless-steel examination tables and tiled floors that are very slippery. The dog can injure itself if allowed to jump. Always help the animal off the table the same way it was put on.

To lift a small pregnant bitch, encircle its front and rear legs with your arms and lift.

FIG. 4-10

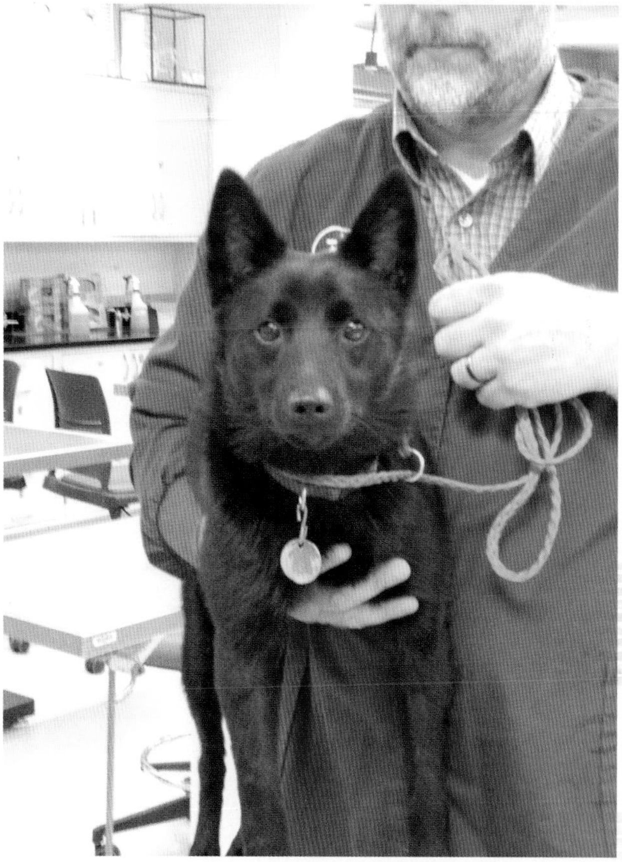

Carry a small dog by resting its chest on your forearm, with your fingers between the dog's front legs for a surer grip. Use your other hand to support the dog's head under its chin, or place your hand on top of the dog's neck to minimize wiggling.

LIFTING AND CARRYING A DOG THAT WEIGHS MORE THAN 50 POUNDS

To lift a larger dog, the two people involved should squat on the same side of the dog. The person responsible for the front end should wrap one arm around the dog's neck and the other arm under and around the dog's chest, behind its front legs. The second person should wrap one arm around the dog's rear end and place the other arm in front of the back legs around the abdomen (Fig. 4-11, *A*). When both people are positioned, they should lift simultaneously, keeping the dog as level as possible. Remember to lift with your legs and not your back and to talk to the dog the entire time you are positioning yourselves and during lifting (Fig. 4-11, *B*).

Though it is difficult to carry a large dog, the best way is to hold the dog with your arms wrapped around its front and rear legs as described previously for pregnant dogs. An even better method is to put the dog on a gurney (wheeled cart) and have one person steady the dog while the other person pushes the gurney.

To lift a large pregnant bitch, it is best to have two people lifting, one person in front and the other in back. The person in back should be careful not to apply excessive pressure to the dog's abdomen, spine, or hips.

FIG. 4-11

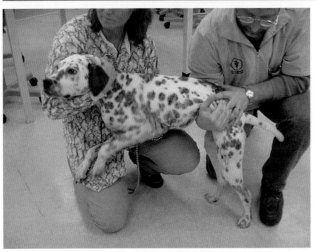

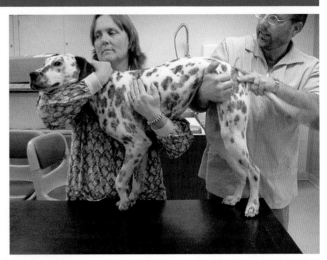

A The person responsible for the front end wraps one arm around the dog's neck and the other arm under and around its chest, behind its front legs. The other person wraps one arm around the dog's rear end and the other in front of its back legs, unless it is a male dog, in which case the person's arm should be placed directly in front of the prepuce.

B Both people should lift simultaneously, keeping the dog as level as possible.

GENERAL RESTRAINT PROCEDURES

Most dogs can be lifted onto an examination table so the veterinarian can perform whatever procedures are necessary. Once on the table, most dogs feel more comfortable if they are allowed to sit. Some dogs are very unstable if made to stand on a slippery examination tabletop. Whether you allow the dog to stand or rest in sternal recumbency will be determined by the procedure being administered.

STANDING RESTRAINT

This hold can be done on an examination table or on the floor for extra-large dogs. Wrap one arm around the dog's neck to control its head, and keep it pressed close to your shoulder. Place the other arm under its abdomen to maintain the dog in a standing position close to your body (Fig. 4-12, *A*). Keeping the dog close to your body and at the edge of the table closest to you gives you maximum control over the dog. If held at arm's length away from you, there is little chance of keeping the dog under control. If you have a very small dog, lift it into your arms and snug it close. This hold is used for physical examinations including tests for temperature, pulse, and respiration (Fig. 4-12, *B*). You can also use this hold to administer subcutaneous and intramuscular injections (Fig. 4-12, *C*), as well as to express anal glands, administer enemas, and examine the animal's limbs (Fig. 4-12, *D*).

FIG. 4-12

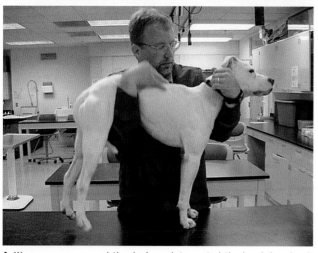

A Wrap one arm around the dog's neck to control the head, keeping it pressed close to your shoulder. Place your other arm under the abdomen, to maintain the dog in a standing position and close to your body.

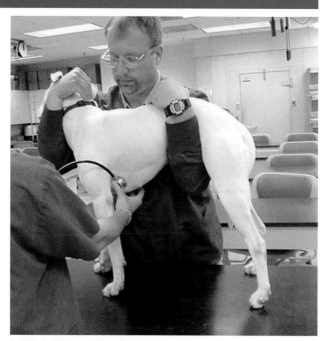

B This hold is used for physical examinations, including those used to test temperature, pulse, and respiration.

(**Figure 4-12,** continued on following page)

FIG. 4-12 cont.

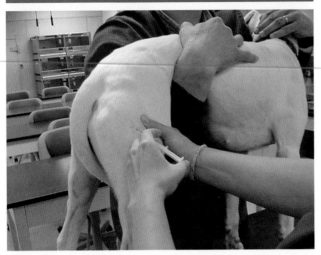

C It is also used for administering subcutaneous and intramuscular injections.

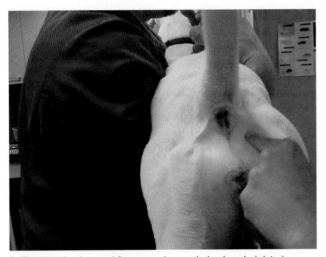

D This hold is also used for expressing anal glands, administering enemas, and examining the limbs.

For rectal examinations, instead of placing your hands under the abdomen, grasp the tail near its base and hold it up out of the way (Fig. 4-13). With dogs of normal weight, you can support some of their weight with the tail as long as you do not fully lift the dog's rear end by the tail. Be prepared to adjust your grasp on the tail, as the veterinarian may want to hold the tail during the rectal examination. You can then support the hindquarters as mentioned earlier.

FIG. 4-13

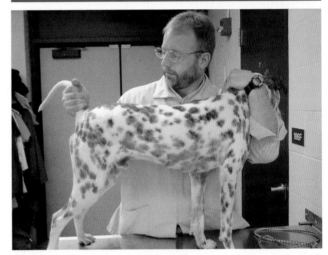

For rectal examinations, instead of placing your hands between the dog's back legs, grasp the dog's tail near its base and hold it up out of the way.

STERNAL RESTRAINT

Begin with proper standing restraint. Maintain your arm around the dog's neck, remove the arm from under the abdomen, and place it behind the stifles (Fig. 4-14, *A*). Gently push forward at the stifles while tilting the dog's neck back. This causes the back legs to buckle and the dog will sit (Fig. 4-14, *B*). Position the dog against your shoulder and body to maintain control of the animal (Fig. 4-14, *C*). Maintain control of the dog's head with one arm while bringing your other arm over the animal's body and grasping its front limbs with that hand. Place your finger between the dog's legs to give you added control. Simultaneously use your arm and body to gently push on the dog's back while slowly pulling its front legs forward to guide the dog into the sternal position (Fig. 4-14, *D*). Maintain the animal in sternal position by keeping one arm around its neck and the other either around its rear or over its side. Keep the dog's body pressed up against yours for added control.

FIG. 4-14

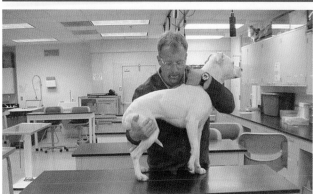

A Maintain your arm around the dog's neck; remove the arm from under the abdomen and place it behind the stifles.

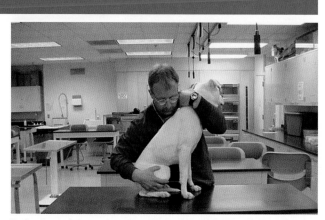

B Gently push forward at the stifles, while tilting the dog's neck back. This causes its back legs to buckle and the dog will sit.

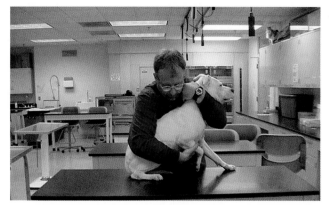

C Position the dog against your shoulder and body to maintain control of the animal.

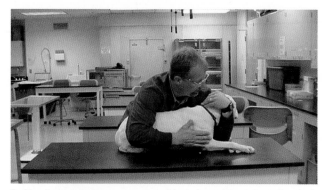

D Simultaneously use your arm and body to gently push on the dog's back while slowly pulling its front legs forward to guide the dog into the sternal position.

Note that the position of your arms may have to be adjusted to facilitate some examinations. For dogs with pendulous ears, pull up the pinna (earflap) and position it out of the way so that you can treat or examine the dog's ear. You can tuck the ear over the dog's head and between it and your body (Fig. 4-15, *A*). When medicating a dog's eyes, simply turn its head so the intended eye is toward the person administering the medication. Sometimes it is best to hold onto the head with both hands, but usually a hand around the muzzle is sufficient restraint (Fig. 4-15, *B*). See the discussion of hand muzzles presented later on in this chapter. When giving oral medication, the restrainer can elevate the animal's head (Fig. 4-15, *C*).

FIG. 4-15

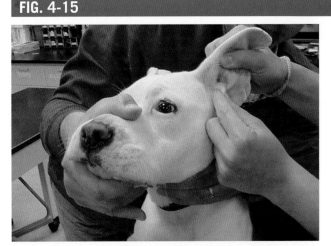

A You can tuck the dog's ear over its head and between it and your body.

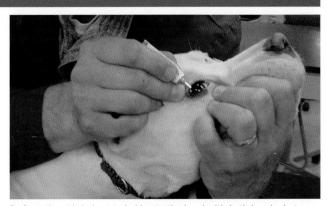

B Sometimes it is best to hold onto the head with both hands, but usually a hand around the muzzle is sufficient restraint.

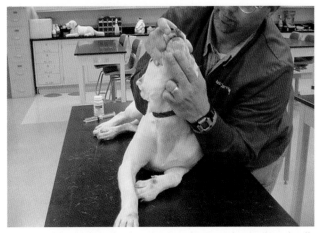

C When giving oral medication, the restrainer can elevate the animal's head.

Two people may be necessary to hold large dogs on the table. One person holds the dog around its neck with one arm while draping the other arm over the dog's shoulders and grasping the animal's front leg. The other person enfolds the dog's rear end in each arm to keep the dog in the sternal position and to keep it from leaning over (Fig. 4-16).

LATERAL RESTRAINT

Begin with the dog in standing restraint by holding its head with your left hand. The dog will end up in left-lateral recumbency (Fig. 4-17, *A*). Move your left arm over the dog's neck to reach between its front legs and grasp its front left leg. This action moves the dog's head to your body with your left forearm (Fig. 4-17, *B*).

FIG. 4-16

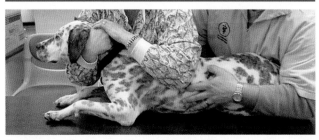

One person holds the animal around its neck with one arm and uses the other to drape over the animal's shoulders and grasp the animal's front leg. The other person enfolds the rear end in each arm to keep the dog in the sternal position and keep it from leaning over.

FIG. 4-17

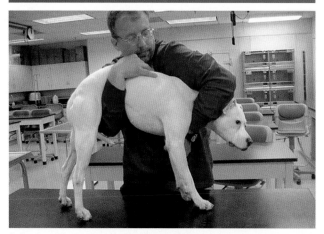

A Begin with the dog in standing restraint with its head by your left hand. The dog will end up in left-lateral recumbency.

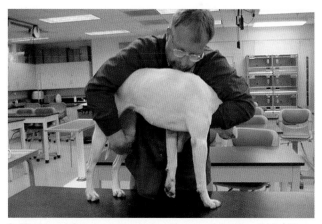

B Move your left arm over the dog's neck, to reach between its front legs, and grasp its front left leg.

(**Figure 4-17**, continued on following page)

Move your right arm over its back, reaching for the left hind leg (Fig. 4-17, *C*). Lift the dog's legs, moving them away from you as you slide the dog's body against your torso, allowing the dog to come to a rest on its side (Fig. 4-17, *D*). Hold the dog down using your left forearm to press on its neck, and that hand holds its front legs (Fig. 4-17, *E*). Place your right arm behind the dog's rear end and hold onto its rear legs (Fig. 4-17, *F*).

The dog's front legs should be held up slightly from the table. This moves the dog to rest on its shoulder and prevents it from trying to stand up. This is especially important if the restrainer needs to release the rear legs for catheterization or to occlude the lateral saphenous or femoral veins.

Fig. 4-17, *E* and *F*, also demonstrates the proper positioning of one's hands and fingers when holding a dog's legs. Placing a finger between each leg provides more gripping power. Note that the hands are positioned above the joints, which provides a fulcrum for the fingers to keep them from slipping down the dog's leg.

FIG. 4-17 cont.

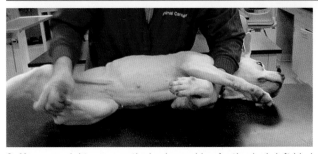

C Move your right arm over the back, reaching for the dog's left hind leg.

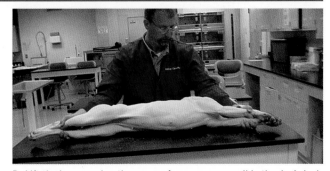

D Lift the legs, moving them away from you as you slide the dog's body against your torso, allowing the dog to come to a rest on its side.

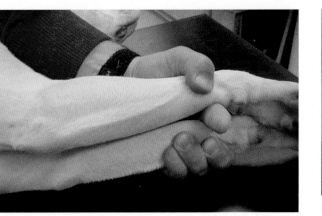

E Hold the dog down using your left forearm to press on its neck, and that hand holds the dog's front legs.

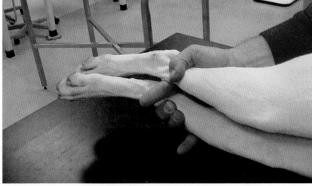

F Place your right arm behind the dog's rear end and hold onto its rear legs.

This technique is also used for a variety of procedures: urine catheterization; nail trims; subcutaneous, intramuscular, and intracardiac injections; or to access the lateral saphenous vein for venipunctures or catheterization.

Follow the same procedure for large dogs, but two people are usually necessary. One person handles the dog's front legs and the other person handles the rear. Once the dog is down, one person can hold its two legs touching the table and apply pressure on the neck and hindquarters with the forearms (Fig. 4-18).

With both large and small dogs, be careful not to exert too much pressure on the neck because you can obstruct the airway, causing the dog to panic and begin struggling.

FIG. 4-18

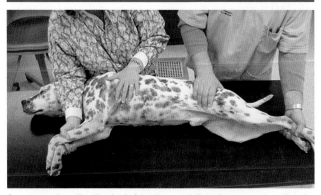

One person handles the dog's front legs and the other person handles the rear. Once the dog is down, one person can hold the two legs touching the table and apply pressure on the dog's neck and hindquarters with the forearms.

LATERAL RESTRAINT TO STANDING RESTRAINT

Once the procedure is accomplished, and if the dog is calm and not struggling, you can let the dog up by releasing its rear legs, then letting go of its front legs.

If the dog is upset, you will want to be more cautious and control the dog's head before allowing it to gain its feet. Release the back legs and place your right hand over the dog's neck (you will have to reach under the left elbow, as that should continue to pin the dog's head to the table) (Fig. 4-19, *A*). Release the dog's front legs, quickly move your left hand under the dog's head, and assist the right hand while holding the head as the dog regains its feet (Fig. 4-19, *B*). Allow the dog to move into a sternal or standing restraint position (Fig. 4-19, *C*).

FIG. 4-19

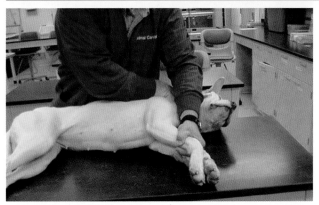

A Release the dog's back legs and place your right hand over the dog's neck; you will have to reach under the left elbow as that should continue to pin the dog's head to the table.

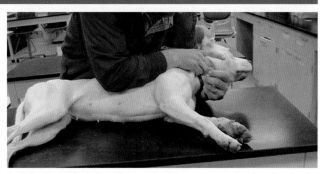

B Release the dog's front legs and quickly move your left hand under the dog's head and assist the right hand while holding the head as the dog regains its footing.

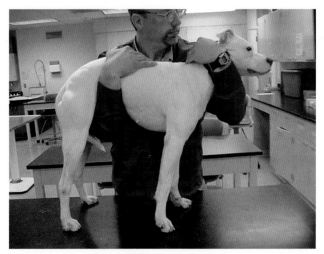

C Allow the dog to move into a sternal or standing restraint position.

STERNAL TO LATERAL RESTRAINT

Place the dog in sternal recumbency, with its left side against your torso (Fig. 4-20, *A*). Bring your right hand up to pin the dog's head to your shoulder. Quickly move your left arm over the dog's neck to grasp its front legs and hold its head to your body with your left forearm (Fig. 4-20, *B*). Remember to position your hand above the carpus and place your finger between the legs. Move your right arm to the dog's hind legs and grasp the left (inside) hind leg (Fig. 4-20, *C*). Note how the restrainer uses his body to keep the animal from standing up. Remember to position your hand above the dog's hock and place your finger between its legs. Pull the dog's legs away from you as its back slides toward your body (Fig. 4-20, *D*). Snug the dog's body close to yours and elevate the front legs, slightly rolling the dog's weight onto its shoulders (Fig. 4-20, *E*). Hold the dog in place with your left arm on its neck and your left hand holding its front legs while your right hand holds its back legs (Fig. 4-20, *F*). An alternative method for a calm dog is to restrain it in lateral recumbency while the restrainer occludes the vessel.

Bear in mind that you often must adjust your hold on the animal because of the animal's reaction to the procedures being performed. Quietly talking to the animal often distracts it during unpleasant procedures. This also can reassure an anxious owner.

FIG. 4-20

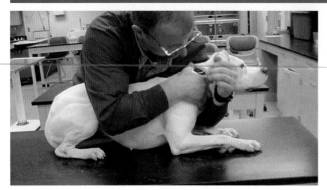

A Place the dog in sternal recumbency, with its left side against your torso.

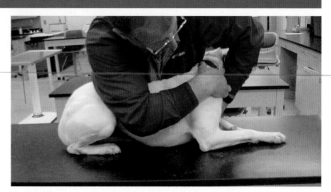

B Quickly move your left arm over the dog's neck to grasp its front legs and hold its head to your body with your left forearm.

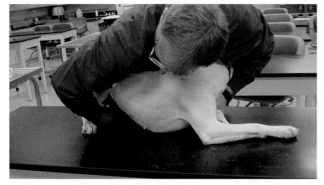

C Move your right arm to the dog's hind legs and grasp its left (inside) hind leg.

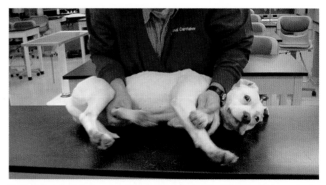

D Pull the dog's legs away from you as its back slides toward your body. Snug the dog's body close to yours and elevate the front legs slightly, rolling the dog's weight onto its shoulders.

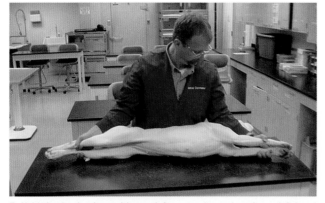

E Hold the dog in place with your left arm on its neck and your left hand holding its front legs while your right hand holds its back legs.

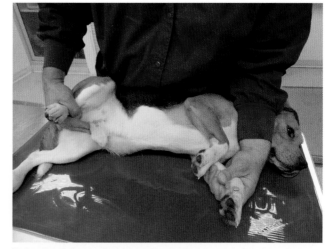

F An alternative method for a calm dog is to restrain it in lateral recumbency while the restrainer occludes the vessel.

RESTRAINING LARGE DOGS

Dogs weighing more than 75 lbs can be handled more easily if left sitting or lying on the floor. To examine a large dog's head, straddle the dog and place one hand on either side of the head (Fig. 4-21, *A* and *B*). If the animal is likely to bite, you can grasp the cheeks or the scruff of the neck. Use your other arm to steady the dog or to help hold it up.

If no corner is available, the restrainer can make his or her body into a corner for the same effect. The restrainer sits with one leg bent underneath and the other leg bent at the knee with the foot resting on the floor. This creates a "corner" when you maneuver the dog between the restrainer's legs. Hold onto the head as previously described (Fig. 4-21, *C*).

FIG. 4-21

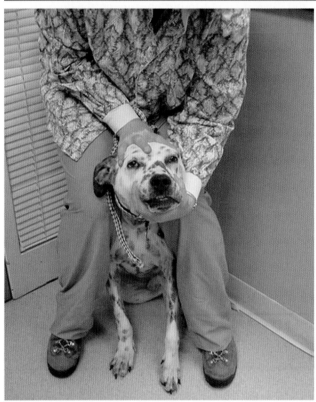

A To examine the dog's head, straddle the dog and control its head with both hands.

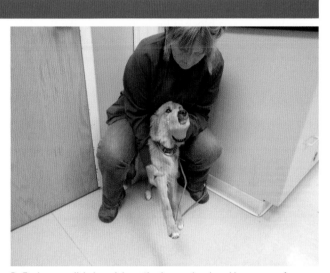

B For large, well-behaved dogs, the dog can be placed in a corner of a room.

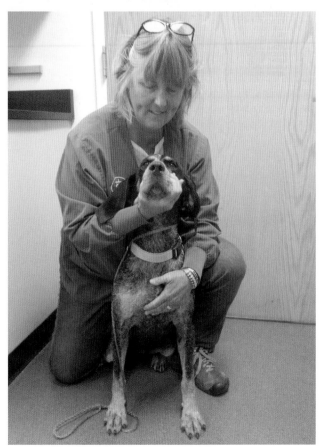

C An alternative is to use the restrainer's body to create a corner.

HEAD RESTRAINT

Restraining the head is very important for medicating and examining the ears and eyes, giving oral medications, and preparing to place a muzzle.

The first method starts with the dog in the standing restraint position. Slide the hand that is around the dog's neck forward, quickly grasping the dog's muzzle by wrapping your fingers around both jaws. Push the dog's head into your shoulder for more stability (Fig. 4-22). Notice the restrainer has placed his head behind the dog's head, using his chin as a block. This helps to stabilize the dog's head from moving back away from the examination.

If the dog is big or hard to handle, you may need to bring your arm from under the abdomen to help pin the dog's head to your shoulder while entrapping the muzzle, then return your arm to under the abdomen. Or you may need to use a commercial muzzle. If that is the case, see the section on applying a muzzle.

The second technique places the dog in sternal restraint. Move one hand up to encircle the muzzle and bring your other hand over the back, resting your forearm against the dog's shoulder; plant your thumb just behind the ear and on the base of the mandible, wrapping the rest of your fingers under its mandible, at the base of its skull. Be careful not to put pressure on the dog's trachea (Fig. 4-23). This technique stabilizes the head for ear cleaning and examination as well as for eye examinations and treatments.

FIG. 4-22

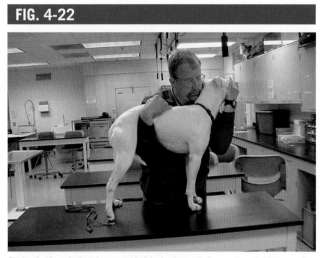

Slide the hand that is around the dog's neck forward, quickly grasping the dog's muzzle by wrapping your fingers around both jaws. Push the dog's head into your shoulder for more stability.

FIG. 4-23

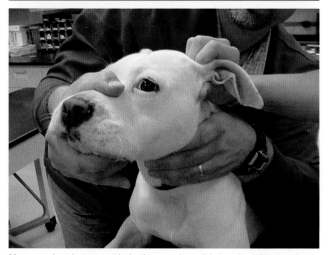

Move one hand up to encircle the muzzle and bring the other hand over the back, resting your forearm against the dog's shoulder; grasp the dog behind its ear, wrapping your fingers around its mandible, at the base of its skull.

The third technique starts by placing the dog in sternal restraint. Move both hands up to encircle the dog's head from behind. Wrap your fingers around the mandible or the ears. Notice how the restrainer leans over the dog's back and encircles the body with his forearms. This prevents the dog from standing up or moving away from the restrainer. This technique is good for applying a muzzle, examining and medicating the eyes, or giving an oral medication (Fig. 4-24, *A*).

If you are alone and have to medicate eyes or ears, the easiest technique is to place the dog in sternal restraint. Move one hand, usually the one with the medication, over the top of the dog's head, and use your other hand to control the dog's head by cupping its lower jaw with your fingers wrapped firmly around its mandible (Fig. 4-24, *B*). Be careful when positioning the tube of eye medication so that if the dog moves you will not inadvertently contact and injure the cornea.

FIG. 4-24

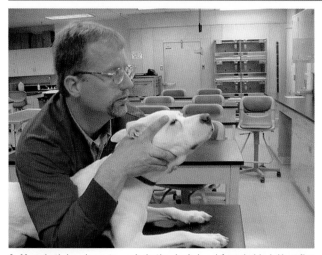 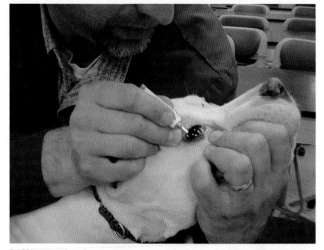

A Move both hands up to encircle the dog's head from behind. Your fingers can wrap around the dog's mandible or ears. Notice how the restrainer leans over the dog's back and encircles the dog's body with his forearms.

B Move one hand, usually the one with the medication, over the top of the dog's head, while your other hand controls its head by cupping the dog's lower jaw with your fingers wrapped firmly around its mandible.

To administer liquid oral medications to the dog, place it in sternal recumbency. Wrap one arm around the dog's neck and lean your body over its shoulders. Use your other hand to insert the tip of the syringe at the commissure of the lips and deliver the medication (Fig. 4-25, *A*). To administer a solid medication, start with the dog in sternal recumbency, hold the pill in the (left) hand, and reach over the dog's shoulders with the (right) hand (Fig. 4-25, *B*). Continue to move your (right) hand over the dog's head and between its eyes to grasp its upper jaw, rolling the lips in over its molars as you elevate its head. Use your (left/pill) hand to steady the dog under the chin (Fig. 4-25, *C*). As you lift the dog's head and roll its lips, bring your (left) hand around to the front of the dog's lower jaw; using your middle finger, pull its jaw downward (Fig. 4-25, *D*). Quickly insert the pill in the back of the dog's throat, following with your (left) index finger to push the pill past the tongue (Fig. 4-25, *E*). Watch to make sure the dog swallows the pill.

You can also use this technique if you need to examine the dog's mouth. By rolling the dog's lips over its teeth, you prevent the dog from biting down on your fingers. If the dog is a bit naughty, you may need a second person to keep the dog in sternal recumbency.

FIG. 4-25

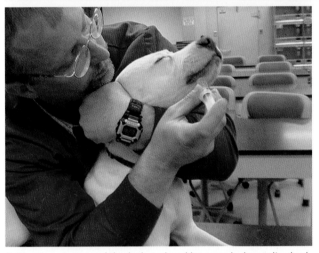

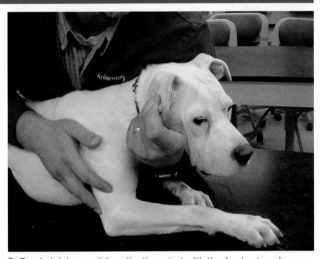

A Wrap one arm around the dog's neck and lean your body over its shoulders. Use your other hand to insert the tip of the syringe at the commissure of the dog's lips and deliver the medication.

B To administer a solid medication, start with the dog in sternal recumbency, hold the pill in your (left) hand, and reach over the dog's shoulders with your (right).

(**Figure 4-25**, continued on following page)

FIG. 4-25 cont.

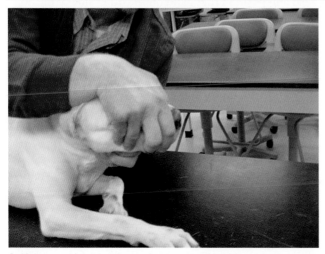

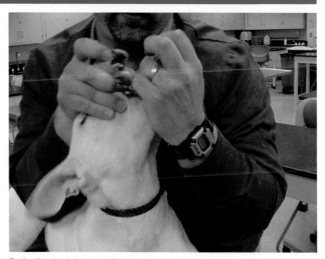

C Move your (right) hand over the dog's head and between its eyes to grasp its upper jaw, rolling its lips in over the molars as you elevate its head. Use your (left) hand to steady the dog under its chin.

D As the dog's head is lifted and lips rolled, bring your (left) hand around to the front of the dog's lower jaw and, using one of your middle fingers, pull its jaw down.

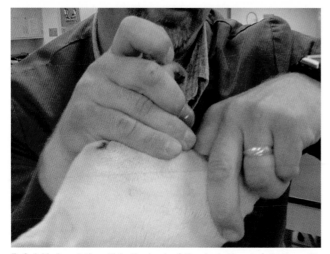

E Quickly insert the pill in the back of the dog's throat, following with your (left) index finger to push the pill past the tongue.

TURNING THE DOG

The restrainer will frequently be asked to present access to the opposite side of the dog that is currently being worked on. Use the following technique to safely turn the dog.

Hold the dog in proper standing restraint. Bring the right arm from under the dog's abdomen to hold its head against your shoulder by placing your hand just behind the ears and extending your fingers along the mandible

(Fig. 4-26, *A*). Remove your left arm from under the dog's head and position that hand on the other side of the dog's head. Once again, grip the dog's head below its ear with your fingers extended along its mandible (Fig. 4-26, *B*). Maintain control of the dog's head and start to turn the dog's head *away* from you, leading the dog by the head, until it turns its body (Fig. 4-26, *C*). Once turned, slide your right arm and left arm into the proper position for a standing restraint (Fig. 4-26, *D*).

FIG. 4-26

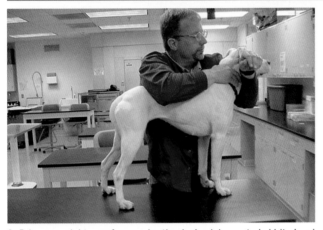

A Bring your right arm from under the dog's abdomen to hold its head against your shoulder by placing your hand just behind its ears. Extend your fingers along the mandible.

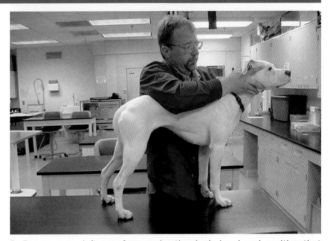

B Remove your left arm from under the dog's head and position that hand on the other side of the dog's head. Once again grip the dog's head below its ear with your fingers extended along the mandible.

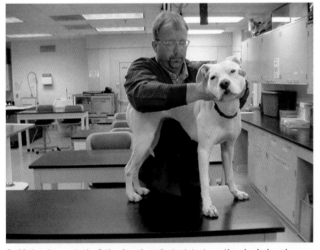

C Maintain control of the head and start to turn the dog's head *away* from you, leading the dog by its head, until it turns its body.

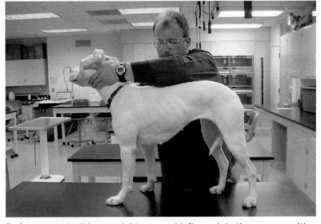

D Once turned, slide your right arm and left arm into the proper position for a standing restraint.

RESTRAINT FOR VENIPUNCTURE

There are three convenient venipuncture sites on a dog: the jugular veins, the cephalic veins, and the lateral saphenous veins. Choosing which vein to use depends on the amount of blood needed and the size and temperament of the dog. If only a small amount of blood is needed or a small amount of medication is to be injected intravenously, the cephalic veins work well.

If a large amount of blood is needed or a large amount of medication must be given quickly, such as intravenous fluids, the jugular veins are usually best. The lateral saphenous veins are usually used as backup veins if the other veins are not accessible.

During restraint for venipuncture, the technician's job involves more than keeping the animal still. You will also be expected to occlude the blood vessel so it stands out and can be seen and to apply gentle pressure to the venipuncture site after the needle has been withdrawn to stop bleeding.

Venipuncture can be stressful for both the animal and the venipuncturist, so it is the handler's job to calm the animal with petting and soothing words. This helps relieve the animal's anxiety.

JUGULAR VENIPUNCTURE

The jugular veins run parallel and lateral to the trachea. This requires the neck to be presented to the venipuncturist.

Remove the collar and leash from around the dog's neck (Fig. 4-27, *A*). Move the dog as close to the end of the table as possible. Place the dog in sternal recumbency and move the hand that is restraining the dog's head so it is under the mandible, curling the fingers around the mandible. Tilt the dog's head back so its nose is pointing toward the ceiling and slightly toward your shoulder. Bring your other hand around the shoulders to help keep the dog in sternal recumbency and grasp its front feet to keep them from pawing at the venipuncturist (Fig. 4-27, *B*). This exposes the neck for the venipuncturist to access the jugular veins.

FIG. 4-27

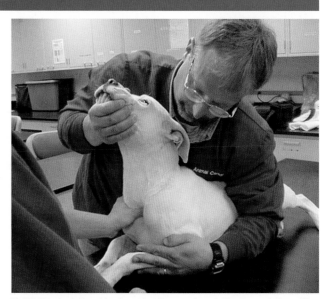

A Remove the collar and leash from around the dog's neck.

B Tilt the dog's head back so that its nose is pointing toward the ceiling and slightly toward your shoulder. Bring your other hand around the dog's shoulders to help keep the dog in sternal recumbency and grasp its front feet to keep them from pawing at the venipuncturist.

With a well-behaved medium-sized to large dog, place the dog in a sitting position either on the examination table or the floor. Use your left hand to reach around its neck and grasp its head to elevate it, and use your right hand to keep the dog from raising its front legs. Many dogs do not seem to object to this position as much as they do to the traditional hold. Use this technique only if you are tall enough to maintain good control of the dog's head. This technique can be used for small dogs if they are brought to the edge of the table to allow maneuvering the syringe. Often you will have to pull their front legs over the edge of the table to expose the neck and have room to maneuver the syringe (Fig. 4-28, *A*). With long-eared dogs, you may have to tuck the ear over the dog's head and hold it in place with your shoulder and/or chin (Fig. 4-28, *B*). Be prepared to switch hands and offer the other side of the neck if asked to do so (Fig. 4-28, *C*).

FIG. 4-28

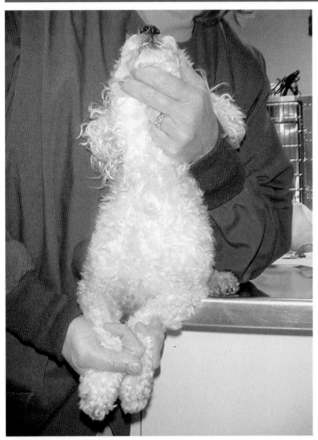

A Often you will have to pull a dog's front legs over the edge of the table to expose its neck and have room to maneuver the syringe.

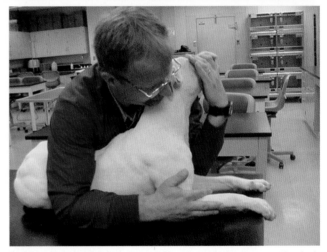

B With long-eared dogs, you may have to tuck the ear over the dog's head and hold it in place with your shoulder and/or chin.

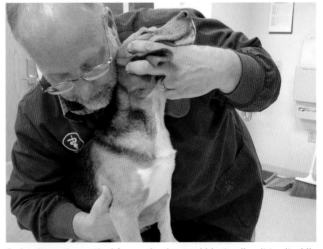

C An alternative method for a calm dog would be to allow it to sit while drawing jugular blood.

CEPHALIC VENIPUNCTURE

The cephalic vein is located on the cranial (dorsal) surface of the front leg. The following instructions are for a left cephalic venipuncture; you should be able to turn the dog and hold it in a similar manner for the right cephalic. (See Turning the Dog for instructions.) Place the dog in sternal restraint so that the dog's left side is away from the restrainer and the front legs are at the end of the table. If you keep the dog's body close to yours, it will help to keep it from wiggling away. Encircle the dog's head with the right arm and turn it away from your partner. Place your left hand behind the dog's left elbow so it sits in your palm and extend the leg out. Ask your partner to grasp the dog's paw and help keep its leg extended (Fig. 4-29, *A*).

The restrainer occludes the vessel by placing the thumb on the medial aspect of the dog's limb, closing down with the thumb and rolling the hand laterally (Fig. 4-29, *B*). The thumb should be perpendicular to the vessel and should apply enough pressure to make the vein stand up. Maintain thumb pressure until your partner tells you it is okay to release the pressure. It is important to keep the elbow in your palm and the leg extended until the procedure is accomplished (Fig. 4-29, *C*). Before the needle is withdrawn, the partner may place a cotton ball over the insertion point and ask you to hold it in place. This is easily accomplished with the thumb. Repeat the same steps for the right cephalic; just turn the dog and use your right hand to extend the dog's leg and occlude the vessel (Fig. 4-29, *D*). Note that you can use this same hold to facilitate nail trims on the front leg; just omit the occlusion of the vessel. Large, well-behaved dogs can be sat in a corner. The restrainer must maintain head control while occluding the vessel (Fig. 4-29, *E*).

FIG. 4-29

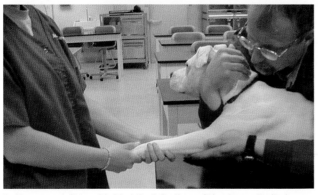

A Place your left hand behind the left elbow of the dog so it sits in your palm and extend the leg out. Ask your partner to grasp the paw and help keep the leg extended.

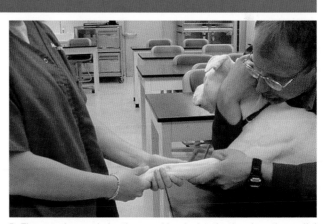

B The restrainer occludes the vessel by placing the thumb on the medial aspect of the limb, closing down with the thumb and rolling the hand laterally.

(**Figure 4-29,** continued on following page)

FIG. 4-29 cont.

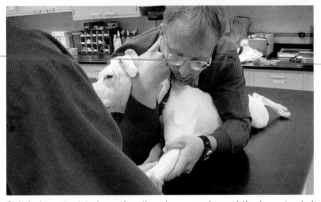

C It is important to keep the elbow in your palm and the leg extended until the procedure is accomplished.

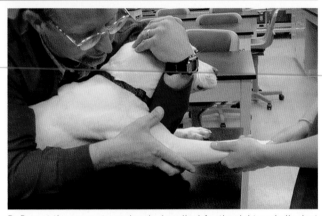

D Repeat the same steps already described for the right cephalic; just turn the dog and use the right hand to extend the leg and occlude the vessel.

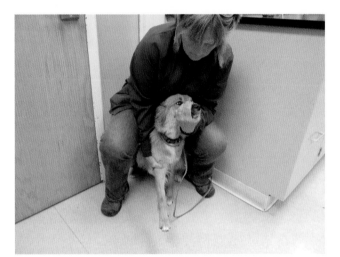

E Large, well-behaved dogs can be placed in a corner.

TOURNIQUET APPLICATION

On occasion, the vessel will not stand up or the dog is too big for the restrainer to effectively occlude the vein. When this happens, a tourniquet must be applied to the dog's front leg to access the cephalic vein.

Use the same restraint technique as described for a cephalic venipuncture with the omission of occluding the vessel. Your partner will gently grasp the dog's paw and start to slide the loop of the tourniquet around the extended leg (Fig. 4-30, *A*). The tourniquet is advanced up the leg until it is proximal to the elbow and then is tightened down. Place the metal clip on the lateral aspect

of the leg (Fig. 4-30, *B*). The tourniquet is tightened by pulling on the straps until the metal clip touches the skin on the dog's leg (Fig. 4-30, *C*). Then each strap should be tugged again to further tighten the tourniquet. It is tight enough when you see the skin bulge up (Fig. 4-30, *D*).

To remove or loosen the tourniquet, grasp the metal clip firmly and push it up as you pull it along the length of the straps (Fig. 4-30, *E* and *F*). It may be a good idea to practice this before you put a tourniquet on the dog. Note that, if you are giving an injection, you must release the tourniquet before injecting. If you are drawing blood, you must release the tourniquet before removing the needle from the vein.

FIG. 4-30

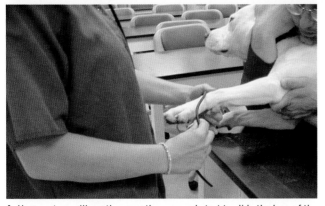

A Your partner will gently grasp the paw and start to slide the loop of the tourniquet around the dog's extended leg.

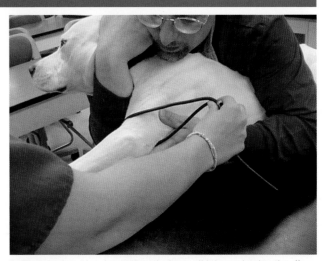

B The tourniquet is advanced up the leg until it is proximal to the elbow, then is tightened down. Place the metal clip on the lateral aspect of the leg.

(**Figure 4-30**, continued on following page)

FIG. 4-30 cont.

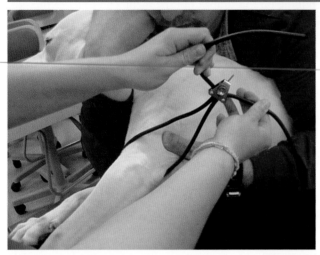

C Tighten the tourniquet by pulling on the straps until the metal clip touches the skin on the dog's leg.

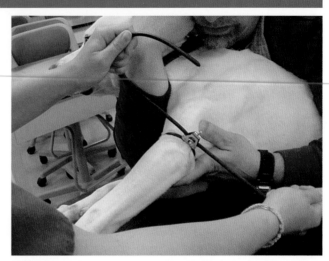

D Then tug each strap again to further tighten the tourniquet.

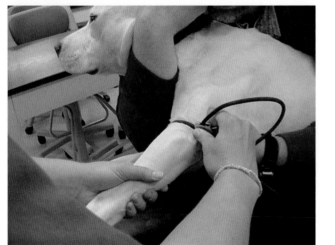

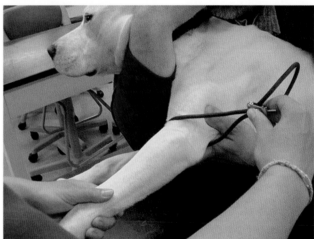

E and F To remove or loosen the tourniquet, grasp the metal clip firmly and push it up as you pull it along the length of the straps.

LATERAL SAPHENOUS VENIPUNCTURE

The lateral saphenous vein is usually used when the other veins have been rendered useless or you must save the other veins for other procedures. This vein curves into an S shape and is located on the lateral surface of the hind leg just proximal to (above) the hock (Fig. 4-31).

Place the dog in lateral recumbency; one hand holds onto the front legs and pins the neck to the table as described previously. Remember to elevate the front legs so that the dog is resting on its shoulder. This will keep the dog in lateral recumbency.

The dog's back legs are released and the restrainer uses that hand to occlude the saphenous vein. Grasp the rear leg in the area just distal to the stifle (knee) joint and squeeze. At the same time, push the leg out to extend it. The person doing the venipuncture must steady the distal (lower) portion of the extended leg.

FIG. 4-31

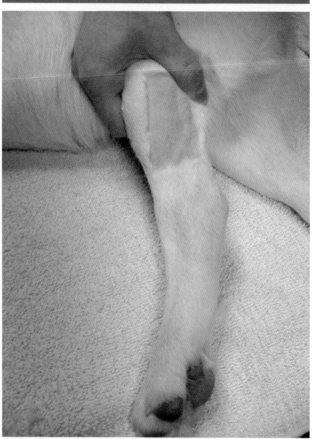

This vein curves into an S shape and is located on the lateral surface of the dog's hind leg just proximal to (above) the hock. Grasp the dog's rear leg in the area just distal to the stifle (knee) joint and squeeze. At the same time, push the dog's leg out to extend it.

RESTRAINT DEVICES

Following is a list of restraint devices and directions on how to use them to help prevent injury to the dog and handler. If used correctly and judiciously, they do not harm the animal, either physically or psychologically.

MUZZLES

There are two methods to muzzle a dog. Commercially available muzzles can be made of leather, nylon, or wire. You can also make muzzles quickly out of roll gauze or nylon rope. Interestingly, muzzling a dog usually takes the fight out of it. Dogs often submit to being handled without much more fuss. However, when the muzzle comes off, the dog may be ready to go another round, so take extreme care!

Commercially Prepared Muzzles

To be effective, these muzzles must be fitted carefully to the dog. If a muzzle is not of the proper fit, "there may be enough play in the muzzle to allow partial opening of the mouth, and thus pinch biting" can occur, or the dog can get the muzzle off by pawing at it with its front feet. Leather or nylon muzzles should only be used for a short period of time. They are designed to keep the dog's mouth closed, which precludes panting or drinking. The wire muzzle, like the type used on racing Greyhounds,

works well because it is designed to cover the entire muzzle of the dog. These muzzles allow the animal to pant and drink, which enables the dog to cool itself. This is an important consideration when handling a dog on a hot day. It is always good practice to keep the muzzle on for as short a time as possible. Be prepared to immediately remove the muzzle if the dog begins to vomit or overheats.

Commercial muzzle placement

Muzzling can be done with the dog facing in either direction. Practice both to determine which is most comfortable for you. Be sure the straps on the muzzle are unbuckled before applying it.

Hold the muzzle in your right hand close to the cheek piece with the strap coming between your thumb and index finger. Place the dog in sternal restraint or in a sitting position. Maintain control of the dog's body and head by reaching over its back with your right arm and holding its head with your right hand, under the mandible, pinning it against your shoulder (Fig. 4-32, *A*). With your left hand, reach under the mandible and grasp the muzzle's other strap. Keep your arm over the dog's body and its body close to yours. Use your right hand to point the nose toward the ceiling. With a quick, swooping motion, bring the muzzle up to encircle the dog's muzzle (Fig. 4-32, *B*). The straps will come up

FIG. 4-32

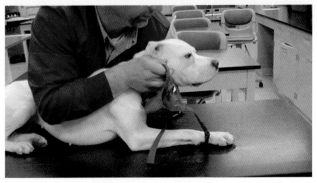

A Maintain control of the dog's body and head by reaching over its back with your right arm and, holding dog's head with your right hand under its mandible, pinning it against your shoulder.

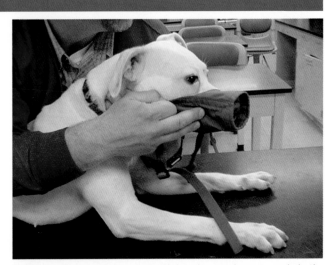

B With a quick, swooping motion, bring the muzzle up to encircle the dog's muzzle.

(**Figure 4-32,** continued on following page)

FIG. 4-32 cont.

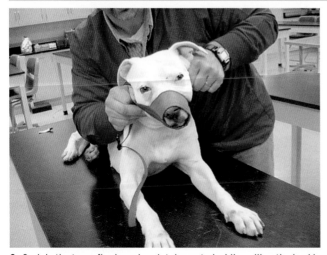

C Grab both straps firmly and maintain control while pulling the buckle behind the dog's ears.

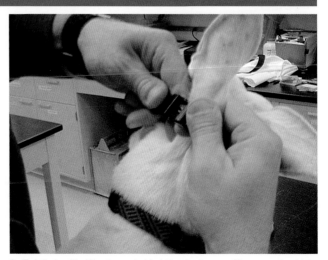

D Tightly buckle the straps behind the dog's ears. The ears should be over the straps.

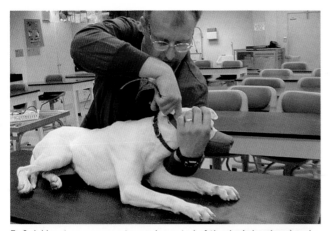

E Quickly return your arm to regain control of the dog's head and maintain the dog in sternal restraint.

on either side of the dog's face. Grab both straps firmly and maintain control while pulling the buckle behind the dog's ears (Fig. 4-32, *C*). Tightly buckle the straps behind the ears. The dog's ears should be over the cheek straps (Fig. 4-32, *D*). Quickly return your arm to regain control of the dog's head and maintain the dog in sternal restraint (Fig. 4-32, *E*). Keep the dog's head close to your shoulder and prevent the dog from pawing at the muzzle with its front feet by holding them with a finger in between the front legs.

Check the muzzle to be sure you can see the dog's nares. If you cannot, the dog may not be able to breathe properly, so the muzzle should be readjusted. Do not put your fingers near the open end of the muzzle; the dog may still be able to bite down.

FIG. 4-33

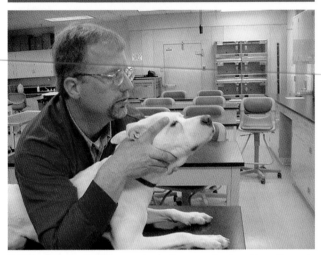

Hold the dog's head still by grasping both ears and excess skin on the neck.

If the dog is extremely aggressive, you may need two people to put the muzzle on. Place the dog in a sitting position or in sternal recumbency. Hold its head still by grasping both ears and excess skin on the neck. The other person approaches from the side, slips the muzzle on, and buckles it in place (Fig. 4-33).

Removal of a commercial muzzle

Place the dog in sternal restraint. Establish good head control by slipping your left hand around the dog's neck. Unfasten the buckle with your right hand (Fig. 4-34, *A*). Grasp the outside strap while maintaining good head control (Fig. 4-34, *B*). Quickly pull the muzzle off the dog's muzzle by pulling forward and to the right (Fig. 4-34, *C*).

Do not move your hand in front of the dog's muzzle as you remove the muzzle. This would place your hand directly in front of the dog's mouth, setting you up for a bite. Maintain control of the dog's head at all times.

FIG. 4-34

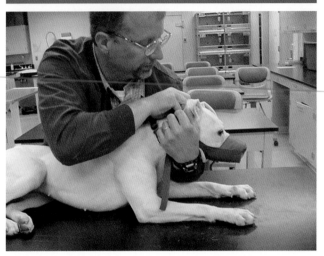

A Establish good head control by slipping your left hand around the dog's neck. Unfasten the buckle with your right hand.

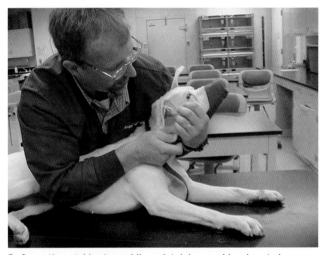

B Grasp the outside strap while maintaining good head control.

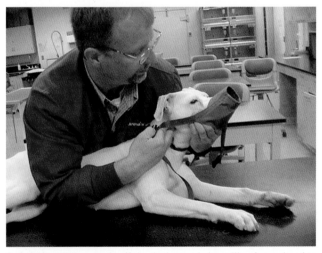

C Quickly pull the muzzle off the dog's muzzle by pulling forward and to the right.

Gauze or Rope Muzzle

This muzzle should only be used for the length of time it takes to complete the planned procedure. The dog cannot pant or drink with the muzzle on and therefore can suffer if it is left in place for an extended period of time. This technique requires two people: one to hold the dog, the other to place the muzzle.

Prepare the gauze muzzle by pulling a "wing span" of roll gauze from the roll for small to medium-sized dogs and two "wing spans" for large dogs (Fig. 4-35, *A*). A wingspan is your arms extended out to the sides of your body. Do not undermeasure, because if the length is too short you will not be able to tie it on properly and your hands will be too close to the muzzle.

Tie and tighten the first of two overhand knots in the center of the length of gauze (Fig. 4-35, *B*). This first knot will hold the loop of gauze open and add weight to the loop for easier placement around the dog's muzzle. Start another overhand knot, but do not pull it tight (Fig. 4-35, *C*). This makes a loop in the gauze that is your initial loop around the dog's muzzle. Make sure the first knot is in the middle at the bottom of this loop.

The restrainer places the dog in sternal restraint. Place both hands on either side of the dog's head, curling the fingers under the mandible for maximum holding and control. Tip the dog's nose toward the ceiling. Be sure both of your hands are away from the dog's mouth (Fig. 4-35, *D*).

FIG. 4-35

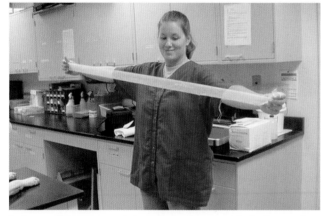

A Prepare the gauze muzzle by pulling a "wing span" of roll gauze from the roll for small to medium-sized dogs and two "wing spans" for large dogs.

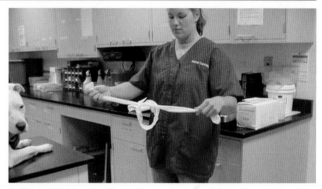

B Tie and tighten the first of two overhand knots in the center of the length of gauze.

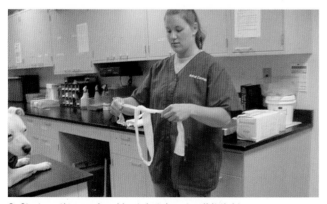

C Start another overhand knot, but do not pull it tight.

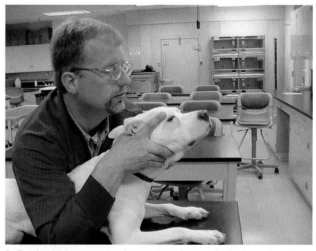

D Tip the dog's nose toward the ceiling. Be sure both of your hands are away from the dog's mouth.

(**Figure 4-35,** continued on following page)

The person holding the muzzle should open the loop up very wide so the fingers do *not* get close to the muzzle. Hold the long ends pinned to the palms. Step up to the dog with the loop held open and start to slide it over the dog's muzzle (Fig. 4-35, *E*). Retain the long ends in your hands as you drop the sides of the loop around the muzzle. Quickly pull the long ends to tighten the muzzle over the dog's jaws (Fig. 4-35, *F*). The muzzle should be tight enough to hold the dog's jaws closed. This is often tighter than one thinks.

The restrainer's job is to hang onto the head. Most dogs will object at this stage and may whip their heads around or try to use their paws to pull the loop off. Quickly bring the ends of the gauze under the muzzle and cross them or tie them with another overhand knot. Bring the ends of the gauze under the ears and behind the dog's head (Fig. 4-35, *G*). Tie a bow as close to the back of the dog's head as you can (Fig. 4-35, *H*). This should be very tight to keep the dog from pawing the loops off the muzzle.

Note that tying the ends in a bow is important because if the animal starts to struggle it can become hypoxic or may vomit. Tying the muzzle with a bow allows a quick release if this should happen. Prevent the dog's front feet from pawing at the muzzle by holding onto its front legs with your finger in between. Proceed with procedures as planned.

FIG. 4-35 cont.

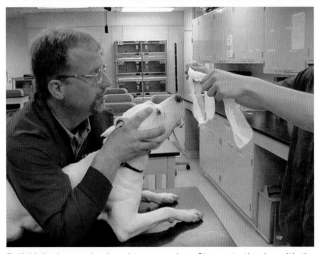

E Hold the long ends pinned to your palms. Step up to the dog with the loop held open and start to slide it over the dog's muzzle.

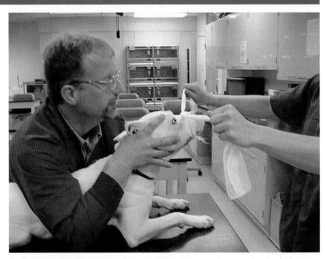

F Quickly pull the long ends to tighten the muzzle over the dog's jaws.

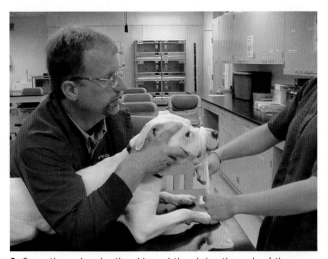

G Cross the end under the chin and then bring the ends of the gauze under the ears and behind the head.

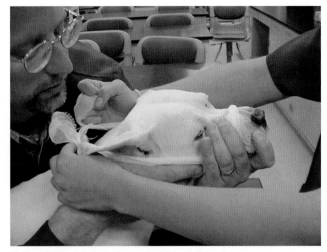

H Tie a bow as close to the back of the dog's head as you can.

FIG. 4-36

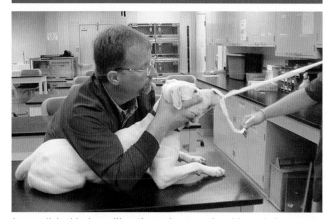

Accomplish this by pulling the end out to the side and then to the front of the dog's muzzle in an alternating fashion until the muzzle is removed.

FIG. 4-37

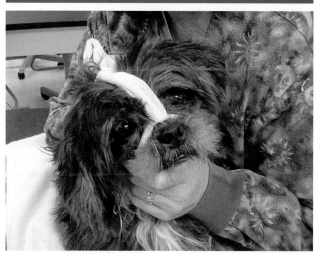

A Take one of the ends down between the dog's eyes and bring it beneath the loop of gauze on top of its nose.

When both of you are ready to deal with an unmuzzled dog, the restrainer moves his hands back to the dog's head with both hands, as described for starting the muzzle. The other person unties the bow from behind the ears and moves his or her hands out to the long ends of the gauze. Then start to "walk" the muzzle off the dog. Accomplish this by pulling the end out to the side and then to the front of the dog's muzzle in an alternating fashion until the muzzle is removed (Fig. 4-36). Make sure to keep your hands at a safe distance from the dog's mouth. The restrainer should quickly secure the dog's head to prevent anyone from being bitten.

A gauze or rope muzzle works well on all long-nosed breeds, but breeds such as boxers or bulldogs require a modified muzzle to keep it on. The muzzle is placed on the dog in the same manner as previously described except in place of the final knot, tie a single overhand throw behind the ears. After that, take one of the ends down between the dog's eyes and bring it beneath the loops of gauze on top of the dog's nose (Fig. 4-37, *A*). Then bring that end back up between the dog's eyes to the back of the neck and tie a bow (Fig. 4-37, *B*).

Note that any type of rope or cord can be used to make these types of muzzles, but the gauze muzzle is used most often because it does not slip as much and gauze is readily available. Be sure to use roll gauze and not a material that is "stretchy" like Kling. The disadvantage to gauze is that

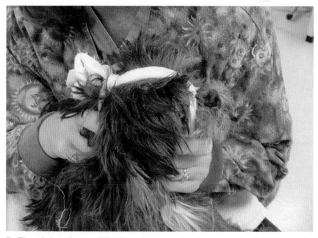

B Then bring that end back up between the dog's eyes to the back of its neck and tie a bow.

the initial loop does not stay as widely open as a loop made from rope, sometimes making it difficult to throw it over the nose of a dog that is fighting.

A word of caution: muzzles are not foolproof. They can slip or be pawed off, or they can stretch, allowing the dog to nip or pinch bite. Even if a dog is muzzled, check the muzzle to be sure it is properly positioned and tight enough before proceeding with a procedure.

FIG. 4-38

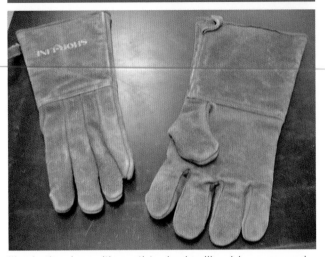

Wear leather gloves with gauntlets when handling vicious or aggressive dogs.

FIG. 4-39

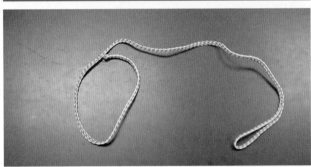

A rope leash is usually made of nylon rope, with a sliding noose on one end and a loop for a handle on the other.

LEATHER GLOVES

Always wear leather gloves with gauntlets when handling vicious or aggressive dogs (Fig. 4-38). The gloves do not completely protect against bites, but they can deflect nips and reduce the chance of serious punctures. Be aware that your sense of touch and pressure is reduced while you are wearing gloves. When working with small dogs (a high proportion of which bite), be especially aware of how tightly you are restraining them.

FIG. 4-40

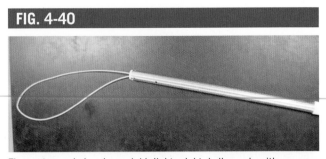

The capture pole is a long, rigid, lightweight, hollow pole with a rope or plastic-covered wire noose at the end.

ROPE LEASHES

A rope leash is usually made of nylon rope, with a sliding noose on one end and a loop for a handle on the other (Fig. 4-39). It is usually used to remove dogs from a kennel or to lead dogs to another location inside or outside of the hospital.

Never tie a dog or any other animal to an immovable object with a rope leash and leave the animal unattended. This can easily lead to accidental strangulation.

CAPTURE POLES

The capture pole is a long, rigid, lightweight, hollow pole with a rope or plastic-covered wire noose at its end (Fig. 4-40). One end of the noose is fastened to the pole and the other runs through the hollow pole. The noose is tightened and loosened using the free end protruding from the hollow pole. The pole should be long and rigid enough to support at least 100 pounds.

A capture pole can keep a vicious dog away from the handler's body and control the head enough to allow safe injection of a sedative. If the noose is too tight and begins to asphyxiate the dog, you can easily loosen the noose without having to get close to the dog's head or allow the dog to escape. It can also be used to maneuver a vicious dog into a cage or run.

A word of caution about rope leashes and capture poles: never drag a dog out of its cage and let it fall to the floor with a leash or pole around its neck. This may fracture the dog's neck or damage its trachea and other vital structures in its neck. If the dog is very strong, two capture poles or a combination of capture pole and rope leash can be used until a sedative can be injected.

FIG. 4-41

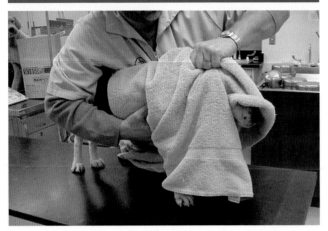

It is best to grasp the scruff of the dog's neck through the towel or to wrap the towel very tightly around the dog so it cannot turn and bite your hands.

TOWELS AND BLANKETS

Towels and blankets work well to remove unfriendly small dogs from a cage. You can toss the towel over the dog's body, then scoop the dog up and deposit it onto the examination table. It is best to grasp the scruff of the dog's neck through the towel or to wrap the towel very tightly around the dog so it cannot turn and bite your hands (Fig. 4-41).

MOVEMENT-LIMITING DEVICES

Movement-limiting devices are designed to prevent a dog from chewing on itself or bandages or to generally restrict movement.

Elizabethan collars are cone-shaped collars that fit around a dog's neck (Fig. 4-42, *A*). They can be either attached to the dog's collar or secured around its neck with roll gauze. These collars are available commercially or can be made from plastic buckets, x-ray film, cardboard (short term), or large plastic bottles. Any material can be used that is sturdy enough to withstand being knocked about or bent, thus keeping the dog from chewing or licking other areas of its body.

Some precautions must be taken when using Elizabethan collars. With a commercially available collar, the main considerations are its length and tightness. The collar should extend past the end of the nose and should be snug but not constrictive around the neck. Homemade collars can present problems because many of them have sharp edges that may injure the dog's neck. With both types, you may have to show the dog how to eat with the collar in place, or elevate the food and water dishes, or take the collar off for the dog to eat or drink. Dogs also often run into walls, doorframes, and the back of your legs when wearing an Elizabethan collar because their peripheral vision is impaired.

No-bite collars are designed to fit snugly around the dog's neck, much like a cervical collar for humans (Fig. 4-42, *B*). The dog is able to eat and drink normally and has full peripheral vision so you do not have to worry about it bumping into things.

FIG. 4-42

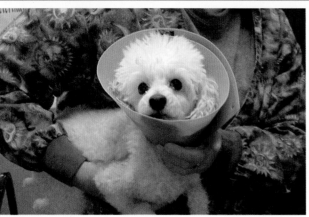

A Elizabethan collars are cone-shaped collars that fit around a dog's neck.

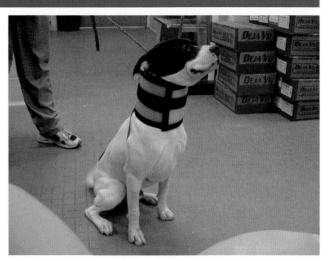

B Restrictive collars are designed to fit snugly around the dog's neck, much like a cervical collar for humans.

(**Figure 4-42,** continued on following page)

FIG. 4-42 cont.

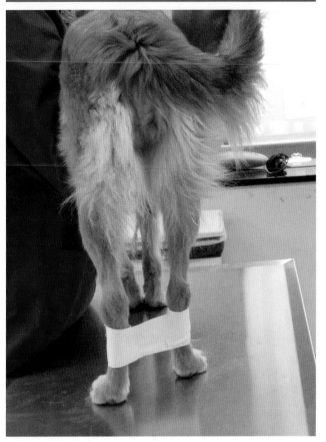

C Tape hobbles help restrain back legs for breeding examinations.

Tape hobbles can be made using wide tape. Be sure to form a nonstick surface by placing the tape back to back. A dog should never be left unattended in this form of restraint (Fig. 4-42, *C*).

SUGGESTED READINGS

Crow SE, Walshaw SO: *Manual of clinic procedures in the dog and cat*, Philadelphia, 1987, Lippincott.

Evans JM: Developing canine social skills, *Dogs USA* 3:64–65, 1988.

Fowler ME: *Restraint and handling of wild and domestic animals*, Ames, IA, 1978, Iowa State University Press.

Kazmierczak K: Bandage management in small animals, *Vet Tech* 3:309–315, 1982.

Leahy JR, Barrow P: *Restraint of animals*, Ithaca, NY, 1953, Cornell Campus Store.

Sonsthagen TF: *Restraint of domestic animals*, St. Louis, 1991, Mosby.

Todd-Jenkins K, Dugan B, Remsburg DW, Montgomery C: Restraint and handling of animals. In *McCurnin's clinical textbook for veterinary technicians*, ed 8, Philadelphia, 2014, Saunders.

5

Restraint of Cattle

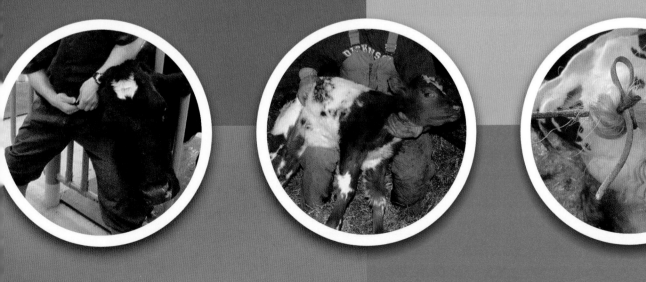

As with all prey animals, cattle's main means of defense is to try to get away from a threatening situation. If they cannot, they will rely on their speed, body, head, and hooves to defend themselves. They will use their heads to push you down or against a fence, which can easily lead to severe injuries. If the animal has horns, being gored is a real threat.

In addition to butting, another defensive mechanism of cattle is kicking. They are accurate with their feet and can kick out 6 to 8 feet from their bodies. The 6 to 8 feet is a kill zone because whatever happens to be kicked can die or be damaged. Most cattle do not usually kick straight backward like a horse. Rather, they usually kick in a slight forward motion that then arcs backward. The safest place to stand is right next to the shoulder or rear of the animal or outside of the kill zone. Be aware that cattle can kick past their shoulders with their rear legs, though the force is diminished.

The type of restraint used on cattle depends on the animal's age, sex, breed, and previous exposure to people. Most dairy cows are accustomed to being touched and having people around them. In contrast, many beef cattle may only see people once or twice a year and then are often subjected to some painful or frightful procedures. This often makes them jumpy and nervous around people. A nervous cow keeps its head and tail up and has a somewhat wild look in its eye. All cattle should be handled in a calm and deliberate manner with low-key commands. This will help them remain as calm as possible.

All bulls, both beef and dairy, are very unpredictable and should always be handled cautiously. A dairy bull's sheer size and unpredictability can kill a careless handler. Signs of aggression in bulls include looking directly at you, pawing the ground with a front foot, and lowering and shaking the head. Handlers should work together so no one is ever left alone with a bull.

HERDING CATTLE

If driven in the proper manner, cattle are easily moved from one place to another. It is best to keep them as calm as possible so that they do not run. Once they are spooked, it is difficult to settle them down enough so that you can direct their movements or accomplish the intended procedures. Urging by voice and proper body positions in relation to the cow's body prompts it to move. A whip, paddle, or electric prod applied only on the rump and back of the legs is used judiciously only on extremely stubborn animals.

Cattle have a pressure point or point of balance that is at the shoulder. Moving past the shoulder going toward the rear of the cow prompts the cow to move forward. Moving toward the head from the point of the shoulder will make the cow stop and then turn to move away from you. Use this information to move cattle into a pen or down an alleyway without a lot of prompting with a whip or paddle.

Do not push cattle too hard when moving a herd or group of cattle into a pen or alleyway. Rather, allow them to look inside and inspect the area. If you do not allow them to look the place over, they will either scatter in every direction or move in a circle and refuse to enter the enclosure. Remember, they do not see well close up and do not have depth perception. Sudden movements will startle them, and a change in light will make them leery. Place one person toward the opening of the gate and one behind the group you need to move. The person in the back puts pressure on the group by stepping forward. The person toward the front puts pressure on the group by walking toward the rear of the group from directly behind their shoulders toward the rear. As the cattle start to move into the pen, the person at the front of the group will continue the forward motion by stepping behind the group as he or she moves in that direction. Notice how the person (Fig. 5-1, *A* and *B*) is putting pressure on the cows to move along a fence. The handler is not following directly behind the cows, but to the side and in their range of sight. This keeps the cows following the fence, and the handler stays out of range of the back feet. The same principles of staying within their line of sight and moving cattle calmly apply to groups of cattle (Fig. 5-1, *C*).

FIG. 5-1

A Notice how this person is putting pressure on the cow to move along the fence. The handler is not following directly behind the cow, but to the side and in her range of sight.

(**Figure 5-1,** continued on following page)

FIG. 5-1 cont.

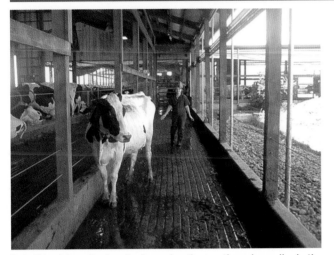

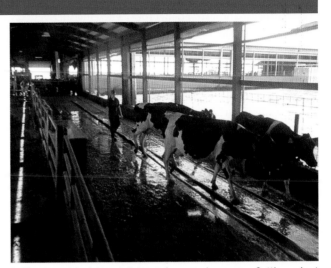

B In this picture, the handler is moving the cow through an alley in the range of the cow's sight.

C The same principles apply to moving cows in a group. Cattle are best moved when done calmly and slowly.

Separating a cow and her calf from the herd is sometimes difficult and often dangerous. They instinctively try to remain with the herd for protection. The best scenario is to move a small group, containing the intended cow and calf, into a pen that has a gate into another pen. One person operates the gate, opening and closing it as the appropriate animal approaches. Two other people are placed in the same positions as described for pushing a group into a pen. Move the mother and her calf along the fence opposite the person at the gate. This allows the gate to close behind the cow and calf (Fig. 5-2).

Remember that mothers are protective of their calves and may chase after you if they feel threatened. Have escape routes in mind, watch the cattle carefully, and never turn your back on the cow or group. Many people have lost their lives to cows that are upset.

It is also important to lock up any dogs that may be around, even if they are trained cattle dogs. A cow with young at its side will get very upset when a dog is in the pen with them and will often charge the dog. Unfortunately, the dog often looks to people for protection and will run behind the closest person. The cow will not differentiate between you and the dog.

FIG. 5-2

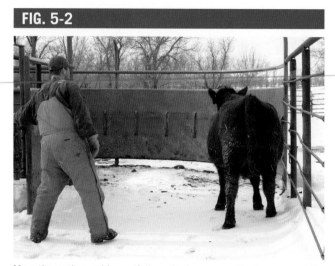

Move the mother and her calf along the fence opposite the person at the gate. This allows the gate to close behind the cow and calf.

RESTRAINT IN CHUTES AND STANCHIONS

A chute is usually used to restrain beef cattle and bulls. The chute is usually at the end of an alleyway that allows one animal access to the chute at a time. The best configuration for an alleyway is curved or a half circle (Fig. 5-3, *A*). To the animal, the chute appears as a continuation of the alley, and the animal often willingly steps into and "through" the chute (Fig. 5-3, *B* and *C*). As the animal reaches the front of the chute, its neck is caught by gates that are closed by the handler or by contact with the animal's shoulders (Fig. 5-3, *D*). At nearly the same time as the neck gate is closed, the rear gate is closed to prevent other animals from entering the chute and to prevent the animal from backing out of the chute. For further restraint, the sidewalls on some types of chutes squeeze in or gates are used to push the animal to one side of the chute. Squeezing the side panels should be the last step in the capture process (Fig. 5-3, *E*).

Some chutes have side panels that fold down to allow work on the feet or sidebars that can be dropped to examine the body or give vaccinations (Fig. 5-3, *F* and *G*). The neck squeeze allows the animal's head and eyes to be examined or oral medications to be administered. During rectal or vaginal examinations, the tailgate protects personnel from other animals entering the chute. Even if the chute has a tailgate, a plank, pipe, chain, or stack of bales should be placed behind the rear legs of the animal to prevent it from kicking the person working on the rear of the animal (Fig. 5-3, *H*). It is important to stand as close to the animal as possible in case it kicks. The kick will not have as much power at its beginning as it does when it reaches its zenith at about 6 to 8 feet.

FIG. 5-3

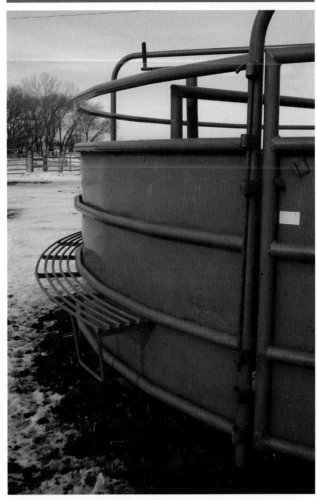

A The chute is usually at the end of an alleyway that allows one animal access to the chute at a time. The best configuration for an alleyway is curved or in a half circle.

(**Figure 5-3,** continued on following page)

FIG. 5-3 cont.

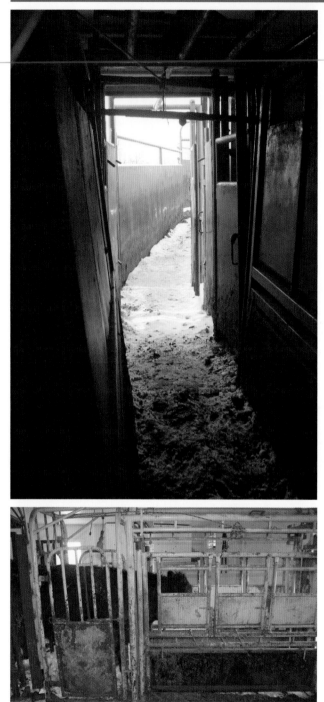

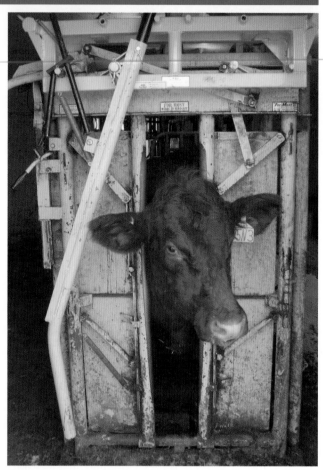

D As the animal reaches the front of the chute, its neck is caught by gates that are closed by the handler or by contact with the animal's shoulders.

B and C To the animal, the chute appears as a continuation of the alley, and animals often willingly step into and "through" the chute.

(**Figure 5-3,** continued on following page)

FIG. 5-3 cont.

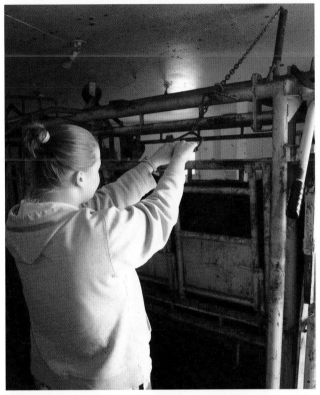

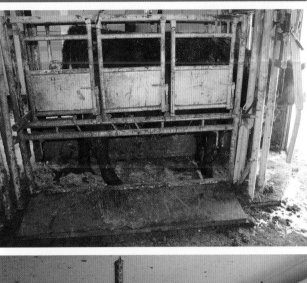

E For further restraint, the sidewalls on some types of chutes squeeze in, or gates are used to push the animal to one side of the chute. Squeezing the side panels should be the last step in the capture process.

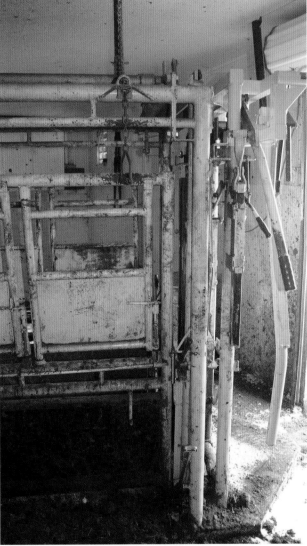

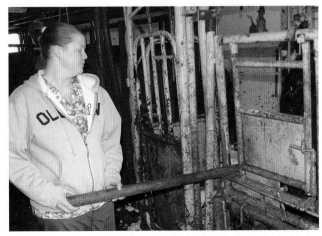

H Even if the chute has a tailgate, a plank, pipe, chain, or stack of bales should be placed behind the rear legs of the animal to prevent it from kicking the person working on the rear of the animal.

F and G Some chutes have side panels that fold down to allow you to work on your feet, or sidebars that can be dropped to examine the animal's body or give vaccinations.

To release an animal from the chute, the operation is reversed. The body squeeze is released, the neck squeeze is opened wide, and the animal is moved out of the chute. Remember to move from the shoulder toward the rear of the animal to get it to leave the chute. Always ready the neck catch on the chute for the next animal before opening the rear gate. This prevents an anxious animal from charging through the chute before you are ready to catch it.

There are many types of chutes. You can save time and avoid injuries if you familiarize yourself with the operation of the chute before using it. Another thing to keep in mind is to make sure the area just in front of the chute is open with no distractions. If a fence, body, or anything else blocks the entrance, the cow will be reluctant to move in that direction. In addition, if the cattle are riled up, they may charge the entrance, so be ready to catch them very quickly!

Most dairy cows are treated in a stanchion. Stanchions are simple head catches (Fig. 5-4, *A*) that usually have a horizontal single bar on the sides and an open rear area (Fig. 5-4, *B*). Stanchions are preferable for dairy cows because, as mentioned previously, most dairy cattle are accustomed to being worked on and do not resist quite as strongly as beef cattle. Take precautions to avoid being kicked or butted. Remember to check the ear tag to ensure that you are treating the correct animal and to mark any samples that may be taken from the cow (Fig. 5-4, *C*).

You can perform many procedures, such as physical examinations, intramuscular injections, and subcutaneous injections through the bars on the side of the chute or stanchion (Fig. 5-4, *D*). You can administer oral medications, like drenching, with the animal in the chute (Fig. 5-4, *E*). See the section on oral medications for complete instructions. You can also treat the udder or perform procedures at the cow's side (Fig. 5-4, *F*).

FIG. 5-4

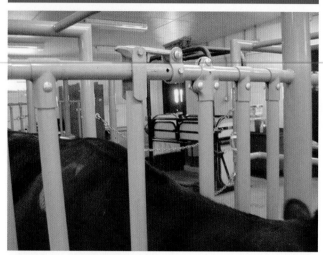

A Most dairy cows are treated in a stanchion.

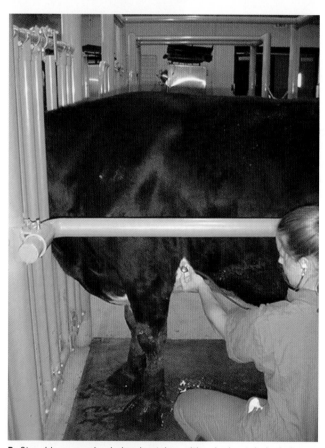

B Stanchions are simple head catches with a horizontal single bar on the sides and an open rear area.

(**Figure 5-4**, continued on following page)

FIG. 5-4 cont.

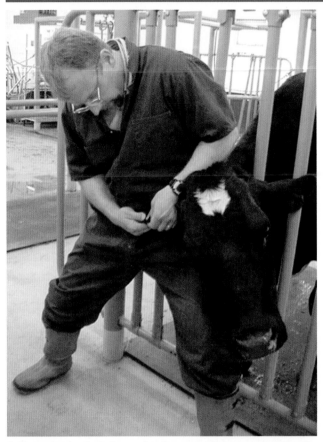

C Remember to check the ear tag to ensure that you are treating the correct animal and to mark any samples that may be taken from the cow.

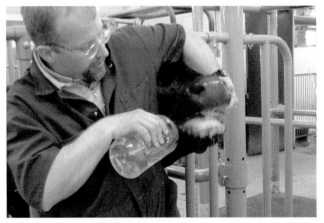

E Oral medications, like drenching, can be given with the animal in the chute.

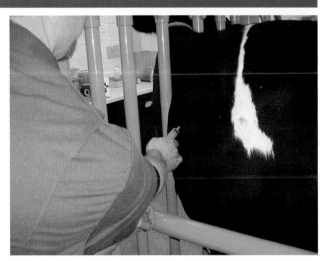

D The stanchion allows easy access to the neck and shoulder area for injections and examinations.

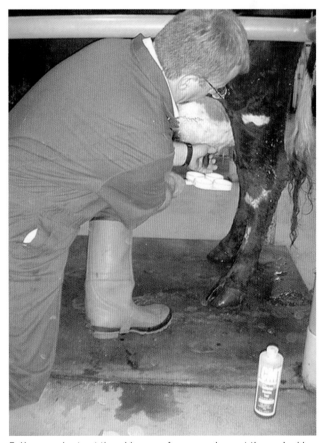

F You can also treat the udder or perform procedures at the cow's side.

RESTRAINT OF THE HEAD

Most head restraint can be applied after the animal is caught in a chute or stanchion. Restraining the animal in a chute or stanchion makes it easier for the handler to catch the head and avoid injury. This is not to say that you cannot be injured once the animal is in a stanchion. Cattle can still swing their heads in a fairly high and wide arc. Cattle with horns can do considerable damage. For this reason, always approach the animal from the side because approaching directly from the front may be construed as a challenge or a threat, and the animal may try to butt you. You will also want to position your body as close to the side of the animal's head as possible. If you are working with an animal that has horns, stand so a horn is behind you, unless a horn curves in toward the head, in which case you can stand behind a horn. Be ready to dart out of the way if the animal should swing its head.

ROPE HALTER

A rope halter is the best tool for restraining the head of a cow. A properly placed halter will not injure the animal if it must be tied for a long period, and the halter is strong enough to restrain the head in different positions.

To apply the halter, locate the noseband, which is adjustable; this should be made big enough to go around the nose (muzzle), and it should tighten down when the end is pulled. The headstall is the longer loop that goes around the back of the animal's head and behind the ears. It is also adjustable, but from the noseband, and should be made large enough to fit before starting to put it on the animal!

Stand on the left side of the animal and place the noseband around the muzzle (Fig. 5-5, *A*), with the portion that tightens under the chin and the loose end coming out of the left side (Fig. 5-5, *B*). Place the headstall behind the animal's ears (Fig. 5-5, *C* and *D*) and tighten it down so it fits snugly. Do not leave the headstall in front of the ears, as the halter could slip off. Check the halter for a proper fit. No part of the halter should be close to or over the animal's eyes. If the noseband is over the eyes, pull it down toward the nose. But be careful not to pull it so it is past the nasal bones because the rope could block off the nasal passages. The animal's head may now be secured for examination of the eyes, ears, or mouth or for jugular venipuncture. Most often the cow's head is brought to the side and tied to the front of the chute (Fig. 5-5, *E* and *F*). Use a snubbing hitch or a halter tie to secure the knot but provide a quick release.

FIG. 5-5

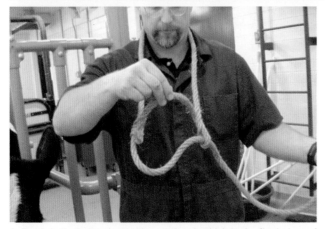

A To apply the halter, locate the noseband, which is the fixed piece of the halter. This should go around the nose (muzzle). The headstall is the longer loop that goes around the back of the animal's head.

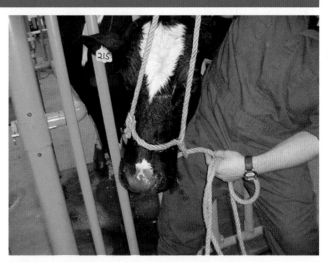

B Stand on the left side of the animal and place the noseband around the muzzle, with the portion that tightens under the chin and the loose end coming out of the left side.

(**Figure 5-5**, continued on following page)

FIG. 5-5 cont.

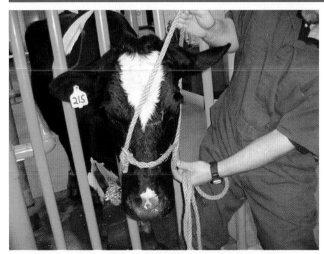
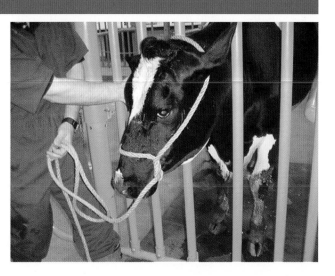

C and D Place the headstall behind the animal's ears.

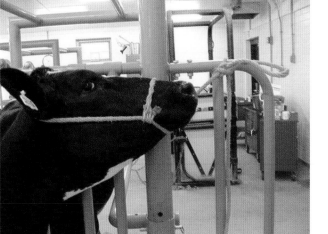
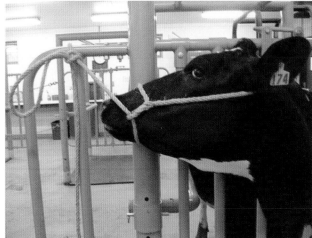

E and F Most often the cow's head is brought to the side and tied to the front of the chute. Use a snubbing hitch or a halter tie to secure the knot but provide a quick release.

If an adjustable rope halter is not available, you can use a length of rope to make a halter. Start by estimating the size of the cow's head, measured from poll to muzzle, and double the length (Fig. 5-6, *A*). Tie a bowline knot to form a loop that goes around the cow's neck. Remember, a bowline knot is a nonslipping knot and will not tighten down (see Chapter 2, Knot Tying). Place the loop around the cow's neck being careful not to get your hands between the poll and the stanchion (Fig. 5-6, *B*). The cow may throw its head and pin your hands between it and the chute. Move safely from the left side to the right side of

the cow's head to slip the loop over each ear. Be cautious as you walk around her head because she may swing her head and hit your hip or shoulder. Do not bend so your face is directly in front of the cow's head. If she should swing her head up and hit you in the head, it could actually knock you out or worse. Pull the loop so the knot is under her mandible, make a bight with the free end of the rope, and bring it through the loop to form a noseband (Fig. 5-6, *C*). Slip the loop around the cow's muzzle (Fig. 5-6, *D*). The knot will be on the left side and the end will be on the right side of the head. Tie the cow so

FIG. 5-6

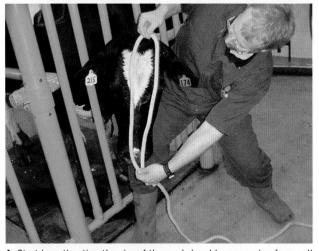

A Start by estimating the size of the cow's head by measuring from poll to muzzle and doubling the length.

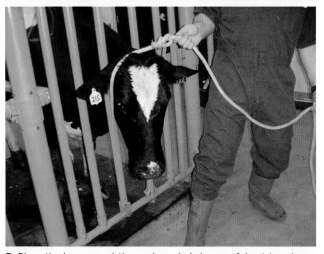

B Place the loop around the cow's neck, being careful not to get your hands between the poll and the stanchion.

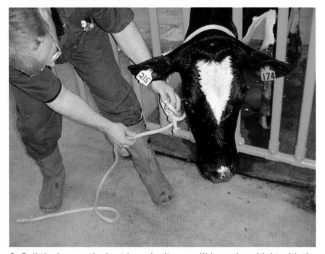

C Pull the loop so the knot is under its mandible, make a bight with the free end of the rope, and bring it through the loop to form a noseband.

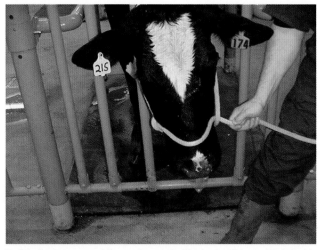

D Slip the loop around the cow's muzzle. The knot will be on the left side and the end will be on the right side of the head.

(**Figure 5-6,** continued on following page)

that the rope will come back over the cow's muzzle. This cow will be tied to the left (Fig. 5-6, *E*). You can make the halter so that the end comes out on the left by starting the muzzle loop on the left side of the cow's head (Fig. 5-6, *F*).

Once the halter is in the proper position and the head is tied securely, you can perform an examination or jugular venipuncture (Fig. 5-6, *G*).

FIG. 5-6 cont.

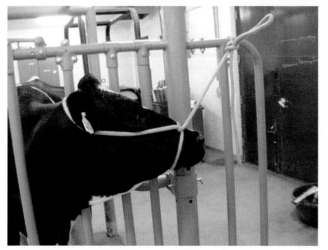

E This cow will be tied to the left.

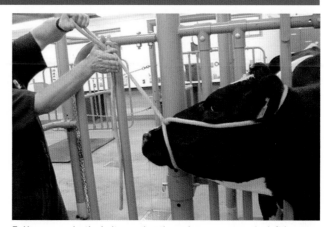

F You can make the halter so that the end comes out on the left by starting the muzzle loop on the left side of the cow's head.

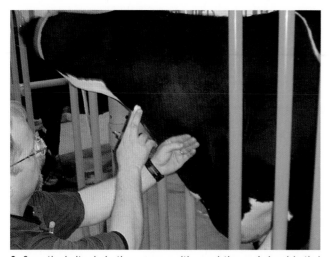

G Once the halter is in the proper position and the cow's head is tied securely, you can perform an examination or jugular venipuncture.

NOSE LEAD

The nose lead restrains cattle by applying pressure to the nasal septum. The nose lead is shaped like a pair of tongs, with a large ball at the end of each arm that fits up against the nasal septum. It is important to frequently check the balls for rough edges because they can tear the nasal mucosa. Also, if the balls are too close or touch each other when the instrument is closed, circulation to the nasal septum is interrupted, causing a loss of feeling, rendering the lead ineffective. In addition, you should never use the nose lead as the only means of restraint. Instead, use it to distract the animal while it is restrained in a chute or stanchion with a halter already in place.

To place the nose lead, stand to the left side of the cow's head, reach your arm over the bridge of its nose, grasp its mandible, and lift up and press its head against your hip (Fig. 5-7, *A*). Hold the nose lead in your right hand so the balls are apart. Slip one of the balls into the animal's right nostril, then quickly into the left and clamp the nose lead closed (Fig. 5-7, *B*). Most leads have a chain or rope attached, so the animal's head can be tied up and to the side for examination or jugular venipuncture. A halter tie, snubbing hitch, or some other quick-release knot is used so the nose lead can quickly be released if the animal falls down (Fig. 5-7, *C*).

The nose lead should only be in place for a maximum of 20 to 30 minutes. The nose lead can damage an animal's nasal septum by decreasing circulation. Moreover, animals that have been repeatedly restrained by a nose lead become increasingly head shy and will violently throw their heads to avoid the nose lead. Therefore it is better to routinely use the halter because of its less traumatic nature and to use a nose lead only when absolutely necessary.

NOSE RING

Most dairy bulls have permanent nose rings placed through their nasal septum. Handlers use two methods to manage these bulls. The first involves use of a bull staff, which is a long rod with a hasp on the end. The rod is attached to the nose ring and, along with the halter, is used to lead the bull.

The second method is to attach two lead ropes to the nose ring, with one person on either end and one handler in control of the halter lead as well. This cross-tying effect is usually considered the safest method of handling a bull.

The nose ring can help control a dairy bull but should never be considered foolproof. Other than chemical restraint, not much can control 2000-plus pounds of excited or angry bull!

FIG. 5-7

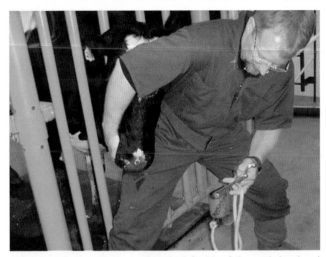

A To place the nose lead, stand to the left side of the cow's head and reach your arm over the bridge of the cow's nose; grasp its mandible, lift up, and press the cow's head against your hip.

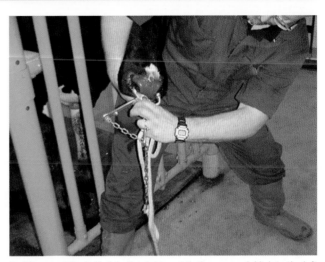

B Slip one of the balls into the right nostril, then one quickly into the left nostril and close the nose lead.

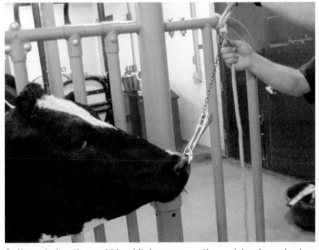

C Use a halter tie, snubbing hitch, or some other quick-release knot so the nose lead can quickly be released if the animal falls down.

ORAL MEDICATIONS

Oral medications are delivered by a balling gun, a drenching bottle or gun, or a stomach tube, which requires a speculum. To open the animal's mouth for placement of a balling gun or mouth speculum, stand to the side of the cow's head opposite your dominant hand. Hold the balling gun or speculum in your dominant hand and reach over the bridge of the cow's nose with the opposite hand. Slide your fingers into the animal's mouth at the commissure of the lips to gently open its mouth by lifting up on the hard palate (Fig. 5-8, *A*). Quickly slide the balling gun or speculum down the center of the animal's throat (Fig. 5-8, *B* and *C*). You will feel some resistance as the balling gun or speculum bumps over the esophageal groove. If you direct both instruments down the center of the tongue, it goes a lot easier. After the speculum is in place, the stomach tube can be passed down the center of the speculum (Fig. 5-8, *D*). If you are using a balling gun, the plunger can now be engaged to deliver the bolus to the esophagus.

FIG. 5-8

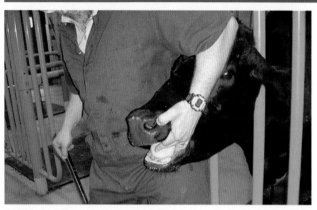

A Slide your fingers into the animal's mouth at the commissure of the lips to gently open the mouth by lifting up on the animal's soft palate.

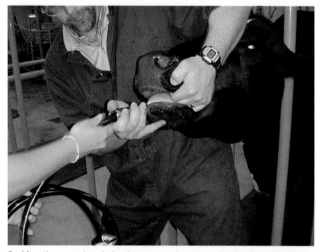

D After the speculum is in place, pass the stomach tube down the center of the speculum.

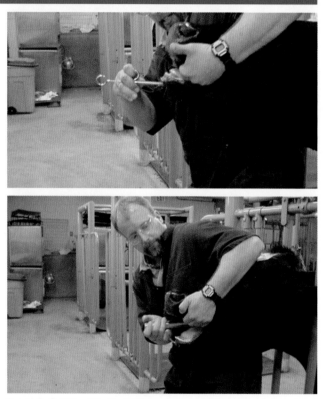

B and C Quickly slide the balling gun or speculum down the center of the animal's throat.

LIFTING LEGS

Restraining the feet of cattle for trimming or treatment of the hooves frequently requires sedation or general anesthesia and use of a hydraulic tilt table. However, if a hydraulic tilt table is not available, you should be able to use a rope to lift feet with the animal in a chute or stanchion.

The equipment necessary for this procedure is a lariat with a hondo. A hondo is a metal piece that makes a loop in the lariat, and many of them have a quick-release feature. The cow is placed in the chute, and for added security a halter is placed and the head tied. This will help keep the cow standing.

Lift the cow's front foot by placing a loop around the leg distal to the dewclaws (Fig. 5-9, *A*). Be aware that cattle can kick you with their back feet, as they can reach past their shoulders. Wrap the rope around the side bar with a half hitch, and then gently kick at the dewclaw area as you pull up on the rope. Once the animal lifts its foot, tighten the rope and secure it with a quick-release knot (Fig. 5-9, *B*). Many cows will kick out, so be ready to take up the slack quickly.

FIG. 5-9

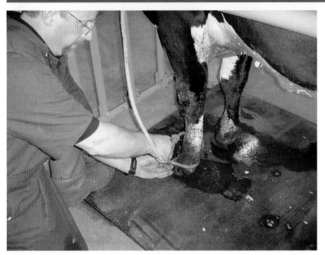

A Front feet are lifted by placing a loop around the cow's leg distal to the dewclaws.

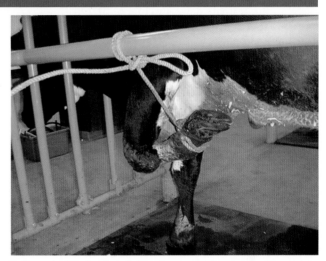

B Once she lifts her foot, tighten the rope and secure it with a quick-release knot.

The rear foot is lifted by placing the lariat over the top bar, using the end of the rope on the outside of the chute to place a half hitch around the side bar. Leave enough rope to tie a quick-release knot when you get the foot into position. Placing the half hitch around the side bar will help to protect your hands when you pull up the slack (Fig. 5-10, *A*). If the cow kicks out, the half hitch will keep the rope from pulling through your hands. With the other end of the rope, place a half hitch above the hock so the end comes out on the lateral side (Fig. 5-10, *B*). Feed the lariat down the medial aspect of the leg.

Never sit when doing this; kneel with one knee up so you can fall back out of the way if the animal kicks (Fig. 5-10, *C*). Form a loop and hook it into the hondo distal to the animal's dewclaw (Fig. 5-10, *D*).

Note that if the cow is kicking, you can fasten the loop with the hondo up high then slide the loop down with your foot or with a broom handle. Pull on the rope that is wrapped around the side bar to start raising the leg (Fig. 5-10, *E*). Pull until the hock is above or level with the stifle, and tie it off with a quick-release knot (Fig. 5-10, *F*). While you are lifting, the cow may start to kick. If that happens, pull the slack out of your lariat as the animal kicks, then tie the rope off with a quick-release knot. Be aware that the animal can still kick that leg out with it tied up. Either pass very close to the animal's rear end or pass way out away from the kill zone.

FIG. 5-10

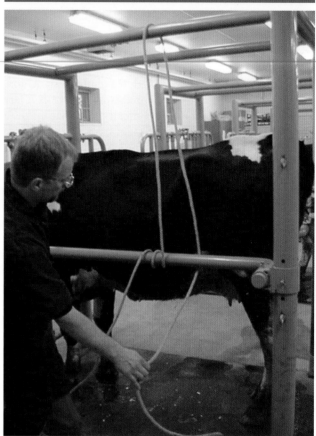

A Rear feet are lifted by placing the lariat over the top bar, using the end of the rope on the outside of the chute to place a half hitch around the side bar.

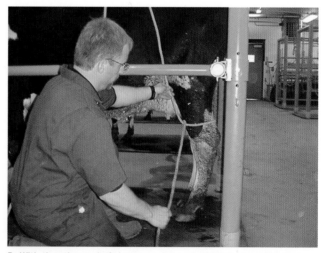

B With the other end of the rope, place a half hitch above the hock, so the end comes out on the lateral side.

(**Figure 5-10,** continued on following page)

FIG. 5-10 cont.

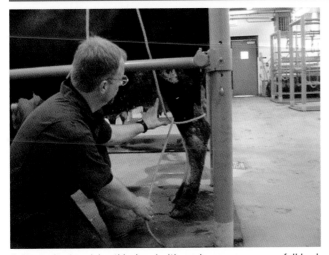

C Never sit when doing this; kneel with one knee up so you can fall back out of the way if the cow kicks.

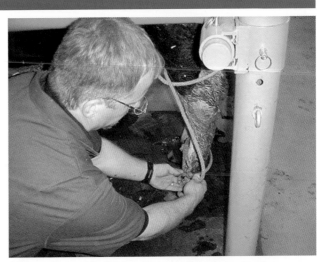

D Form a loop and hook it into the hondo distal to her dewclaw.

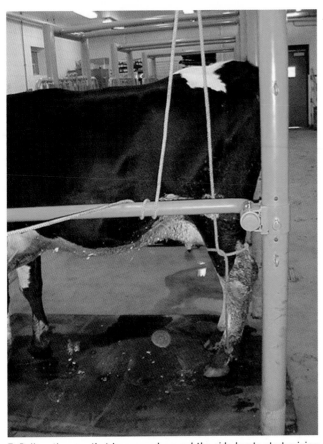

E Pull on the rope that is wrapped around the side bar to start raising the leg.

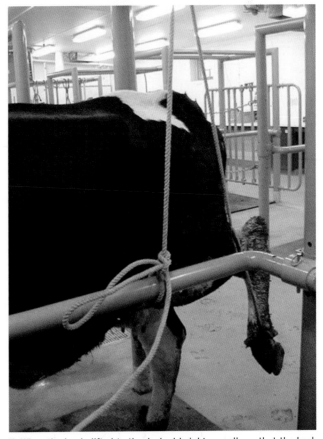

F When the leg is lifted to the desired height, usually so that the hock is above or level with the stifle, secure the rope by using a quick-release knot to prevent injury if the cow falls.

FIG. 5-11

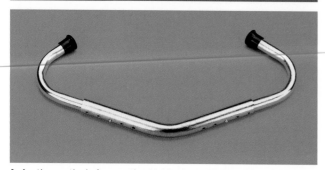

A Another method of preventing kicking is a metal band or bars that are clamped around the animal's flank.

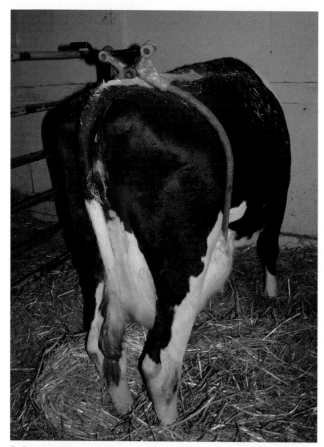

B Position the device directly on the flank and tighten down.

ANTIKICKING DEVICES

Various types of devices are available to prevent an animal from kicking. Milking or chain hobbles have two metal bands that are bent to fit around the animal's leg just proximal to (above) the hock. To apply them, stand on the cow's right side, facing toward the rear. Squat down and apply the left hobble first, then the right. Be ready to move out of the way if the cow decides to kick before the hobbles are in place. The chain should pass around the front of the legs and should be adjusted so the animal can maintain its balance.

A small-diameter rope may also be used as a hobble. Stand on the animal's right side, reach to its left leg, and place the rope around and proximal to the hock. Position the rope so that both end segments are the same length. Cross the rope once between the legs and bring the ends around the right leg. Tie the ends in a reefer knot for quick release.

Another method of preventing kicking is a metal band or bars that are clamped around the animal's flank (Fig. 5-11, *A*). Position the device directly on the flank and tighten down (Fig. 5-11, *B*).

RESTRAINT USING THE TAIL

The tails on cattle are not nearly as strong as that of horses. A cow's tail cannot support the animal's weight and breaks easily if handled roughly.

TAIL JACKING

Despite these limitations, "jacking" the tail is useful to distract cattle from painful procedures done elsewhere on the body. It is also the method used to raise the tail for blood draws.

To jack the tail, place the animal in a chute or stanchion. Step as close to the animal's body as possible so that if the cow does kick it will not be a deadly blow (Fig. 5-12, *A*). Grasp the tail approximately one third from its base with both hands. Use both hands to gently ease the tail vertically (Fig. 5-12, *B*). With the tail in this position, you can perform such procedures as rectal or vaginal examinations, caudal thigh intramuscular injections, coccygeal venipunctures, or udder examinations (Fig. 5-12, *C*).

It is important to keep the tail along the midline and not deflected to one side. If it is deflected to one side, this may make the animal move forward, or you may fracture a vertebra in the tail. When you have completed the procedure, lower the tail carefully. Do not simply drop it.

FIG. 5-12

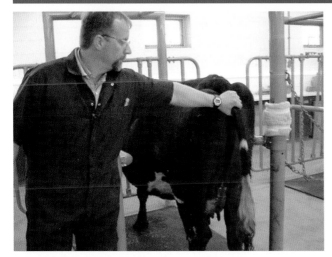

A Step as close to the animal's body as possible so that if the cow does kick it will not be a deadly blow.

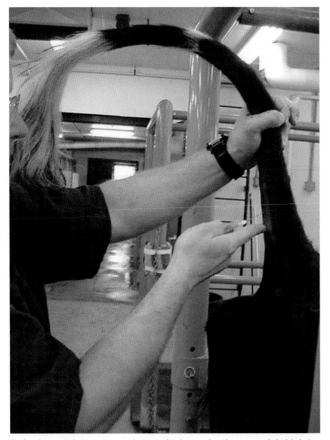

C Such procedures as rectal or vaginal examinations, caudal thigh intramuscular injections, coccygeal venipuncture, or udder examination can be performed with the tail in this position.

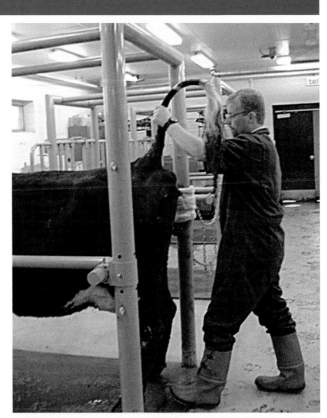

B Grasp the animal's tail approximately one third from its base with both hands. Use both hands to gently ease the tail vertically.

TAIL TYING

Sometimes a cow will swing its tail into your face or keep it in the way as you work near the animal's hindquarters. Tail tying, as described for horses (see Chapter 6) works equally well for cattle. (Fig. 5-13, *A*, *B*, and *C*, demonstrates tail tying in a cow.) Remember to always tie the tail to the animal's own body and not to an immovable object. Tying the tail to a fixed object can result in a fracture or avulsion of the switch at the end of the tail if the animal bolts. Many dairy cows have amputated tails that should not be tied because they do not have a switch at the end to act as the bight.

Some beef cattle accumulate plant fibers or other debris in the switch at the end of the tail. To remove cockleburs and other plant fibers, soak the tail in mineral oil and comb the switch out. Try not to pull too much hair out because this is the animal's only means of swatting flies. The hair eventually grows back if any is pulled out.

FIG. 5-13

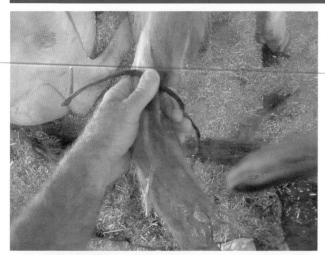

A Be sure to tie to the tail switch only.

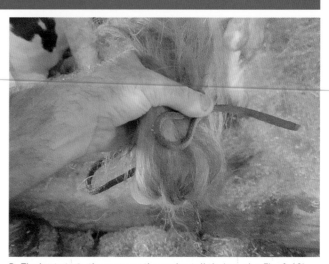

B The knot starts the same as the equine tail tie (see also Fig. 6-19).

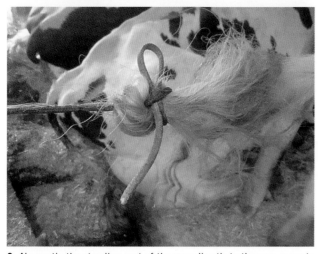

C Always tie the standing part of the rope directly to the cow, *never* to an immovable object.

RESTRAINT OF CALVES

Beef and dairy calves can be handled in much the same manner. Dairy heifer calves should not be handled roughly, as this may result in a bad-tempered adult cow.

Always be careful when working with a calf in the presence of its dam. Cows are very protective and may charge you. A cow can kill a person with a single blow of her head. If the cow is with her calf, move the cow in the desired direction and the calf will follow. Once separated from the dam, move the calf by wrapping one arm around the front of the calf's chest and the other hand around its rear quarters and begin walking it forward (Fig. 5-14, *A*). A larger calf can be led by using a rope halter, but this can often result in a tug of war. It is easier to treat larger calves as adults and simply herd them to the desired area.

FLANKING

Flanking, or placing a calf in lateral recumbency, is easy if you position yourself properly. Place the calf's body so its left side is parallel to your legs. Position your right knee into the calf's flank and reach around the calf's body to grasp the opposite flank with your right hand (Fig. 5-14, *B*). With your left hand, reach around the calf's neck. Lift up on the flank with your right hand and take a step back, letting the calf slide down your left leg to break the fall (Fig. 5-14, *C*). Follow the calf down and place one knee on the calf's neck.

Quickly gather up the back legs and the top front leg and tie them together (Fig. 5-14, *D*). The tie commonly used is a loop placed around all three legs. Wrap the cord around the legs twice and secure it with a half hitch and then another half hitch that includes a bight for easy removal.

FIG. 5-14

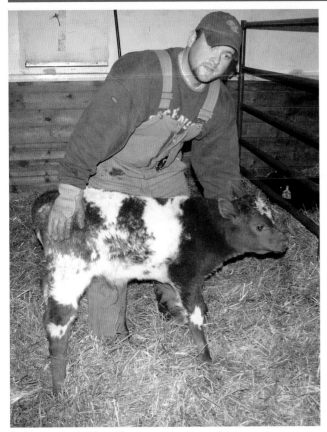

A Once separated from the dam, move the calf by wrapping one arm around the front of the calf's chest and the other hand around the rear quarters and walking it forward.

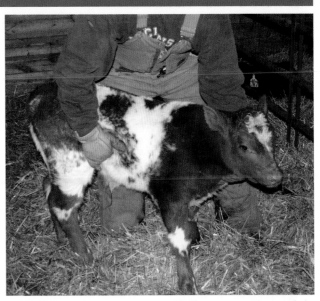

B Position your right knee into the calf's flank and reach around the calf's body to grasp the opposite flank with your right hand.

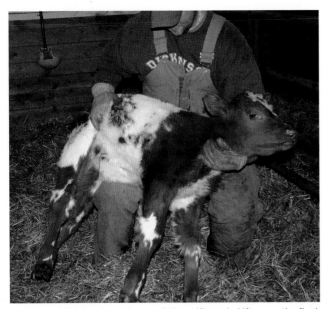

C With your left hand, reach around the calf's neck. Lift up on the flank with your right hand and take a step back, letting the calf slide down your left leg to break the fall.

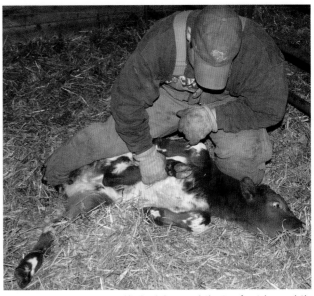

D Quickly gather up the calf's back legs and the top front leg and tie them together.

SUGGESTED READINGS

Aanes WA: Restraint of cattle, head restraint, *Mod Vet Pract* 68: 498–501, 1987.

Fowler ME: *Restraint and handling of wild and domestic animals*, Ames, IA, 1978, Iowa State University Press, pp 113–130.

Grandin T, editor: *Livestock handling and transport*, ed 2, Wallingford, Oxon, UK; New York, USA, 2000, CABI.

Grandin T: *Humane livestock handling*, Adams, MA, 2008, Storey Publishing.

Leahy JR, Barrow P: *Restraint of animals*, Ithaca, NY, 1953, Cornell Campus Store, pp 86–125.

Sonsthagen TF: *Restraint of domestic animals*, St. Louis, 1991, Mosby.

Todd-Jenkins K, Dugan B, Remsburg DW, Montgomery C: Restraint and handling of animals. In *McCurnin's clinical textbook for veterinary technicians*, ed 8, Philadelphia, 2014, Saunders.

6

Restraint of Horses

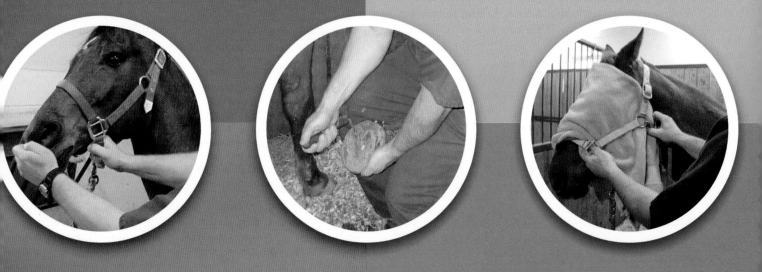

The size, speed, strength, and personality of horses make them potentially dangerous animals to restrain. They have to be treated with respect and caution because they can severely injure or even kill a handler during a moment of inattentiveness. Horses are suspicious creatures and are quick to detect nervousness in handlers. This diminishes any authority the handler may have over them. Most horses are not vicious and most submit to properly applied restraint procedures. Because they have been domesticated for so many years, horses have learned to trust human beings. Most horses you will work with have a close working relationship with humans. Because they are companion animals, it is important to always talk to them in a calm, low voice. This helps to keep them calm and lets them know where you are. However, even cooperative horses can cause fatal injures if they are suddenly frightened or hurt.

Because they are herd animals, horses find comfort in being with other horses and will react if other horses around them spook or get startled. Horses are also prey animals that have evolved a great sense of fight or flight. If frightened or threatened, a horse's natural instinct is to run away, then turn around and see what it was that bothered it—but always to run first. If a horse cannot get away, it will fight to get away. This often causes injury to the handler or the horse.

Horses have keen eyesight for seeing movement at great distances, but they do not see well up close, nor do they see just below their noses or directly behind themselves. Never walk directly behind a horse unless you stay close and talk to the horse so that it knows you are there. Never walk under a horse's neck. The horse cannot see you there and may throw its head, raise a front leg and knock you down, or rear up and come down on you. Horses will run over the top of you if you are between them and freedom or if they perceive you have them cornered.

Horses will kick as a means of protection. They can kick with either back hoof directly behind themselves as well as out to the sides. They can kick with both back legs at once by rocking their weight to their front legs. They can strike with one front leg at a time or rock all their weight onto their back legs and rear up and strike with both front legs. Horses toss their heads, which can cause serious injury if you are not cautious. Never stand directly in front of a horse; it may strike you with its front leg or its head. Horses also bite. They have both upper and lower incisors that pinch, and they can lock their jaws together, making it very difficult to get your body part out from between the jaws. Horses use biting as a means of communication. Horses use nips and outright bites to teach youngsters their place in the herd. However, a horse that bites people should be disciplined quickly and without hesitation.

Horses have elaborate body language that is learned from birth through adulthood. This body language can tell you if the horse is paying attention, understanding what you want it to do, and if it is upset, angry, or in pain. Pay attention to these signals to prevent possible injuries. The most expressive parts of the horse are the ears. By watching their movements, you can get some impression of what the horse is feeling. An alert horse has its ears pricked forward. This shows it is aware of your approach and is curious. A nervous or uncertain horse constantly flicks its ears back and forth, especially if there is activity behind it. An angry or fearful horse often pins its ears back. Do not confuse this sign with the laid-back ears of a horse that is concentrating on a difficult task, such as calf roping or barrel racing.

The tail also indicates a horse's attitude. A wringing or circling tail indicates nervousness. A tail held straight down indicates pain or sleeping. A tail that is clamped tight indicates fear.

The mouth and tongue can also indicate what the horse is thinking or how it is feeling. Yawning or grimacing may indicate pain. When asking a horse to do something new to the horse, you know the horse understands the new task when it smacks its lips or its tongue licks in and out. Trainers often use this behavior as a guide to determine when the horse understands what the trainer has asked it to do.

The horse's eyes can also tell you what it is feeling. If you can see the whites all around its eyes with its head held up and its ears working furiously, the horse is probably very frightened. If the horse's eyelids are droopy or half-closed, the horse may be in pain or exhausted.

Horses can be calmed by an even tone of voice, and most cooperate if handled quietly and decisively. Many horses are easily bribed with lumps of sugar, horse biscuits, or grain. Scratching behind its ears, across its eye ridges, and along its neck also helps to convince a horse that you mean it no harm and want to be friends. Remember that each horse should be considered an individual and treated accordingly.

When properly restrained, you can give a horse injections (Fig. 6-1, *A*), draw blood (Fig. 6-1, *B*), auscultate its lungs and heart (Fig. 6-1, *C*), take its temperature (Fig. 6-1, *D*), administer oral medications (Fig. 6-1, *E*), or perform other examinations safely and efficiently. If you are consistent and firm, the horse will respond to you and try to do what you ask (Fig. 6-1, *F* and Fig. 6-1, *G*). When restraining a horse (e.g., physical examination, blood draw), stand on the same side of the horse as the person doing the examination. This prevents the horse from having to choose which direction to jump if something should startle it.

FIG. 6-1

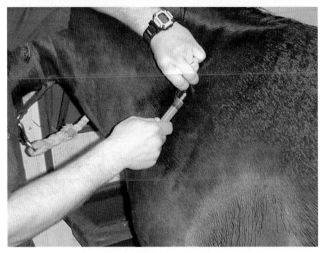

A Once you have properly restrained the horse, you can give it injections,

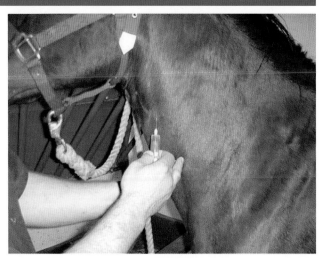

B draw blood,

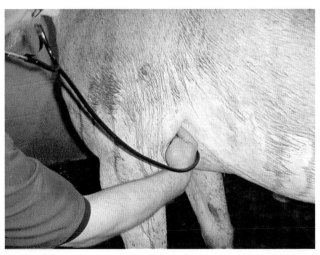

C auscultate its lungs and heart,

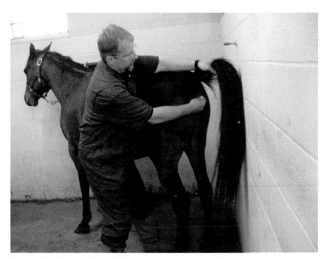

D take its temperature, and

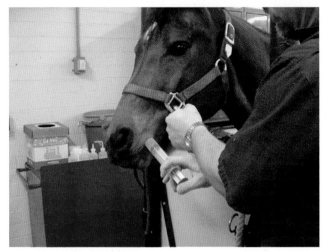

E administer oral medications.

(**Figure 6-1**, continued on following page)

FIG. 6-1 cont.

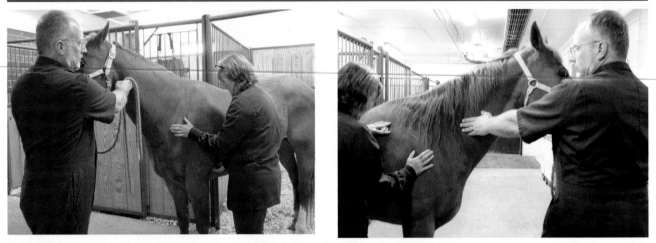

F and G When restraining a horse, stand on the same side of the horse as the person doing the examination.

APPROACHING AND CAPTURING A HORSE

Horses should be approached from the front and slightly to the near (left) side. The reason for approaching from the near side is that horses are accustomed to being handled from that side. They are trained to be saddled and mounted from the near side (Fig. 6-2, *A*). The animal may become nervous if you approach or work on the far (right) side. You also need to stay within the horse's range of vision. Each eye is placed on the very edge of its head, allowing the horse to see straight forward and around to its hindquarter almost in a perfect half circle. A horse does not see directly in front of it, where it would have to cross, or directly behind its hindquarters.

As you approach the horse, watch it carefully. Determine the animal's behavior by looking at its body language and the positions of the ears, tail, and legs. Check out the escape routes within the pen in case the horse becomes frightened or aggressive. If it starts to move away, stop and talk to it and maybe offer it some grain. If you keep moving toward the horse, it may think it is in danger and try to flee. Move slowly and without sudden movements, as horses are easily startled.

Once close enough to touch the animal, it is often best to scratch it behind the ears and on the side of the neck before applying a halter. After this introduction, slip the lead rope over the horse's neck and catch the end as it comes into your reach; tie a single overhand knot to keep the rope from slipping off (Fig. 6-2, *B*). Most horses believe they are caught and stand peacefully, but be alert for the possibility that something may frighten the horse, causing it to bolt. If this happens, a quick hand on the rope looped around the horse's neck and some gentle talking should calm it down. If the horse panics and begins resisting restraint, it is better to let it go than to be injured trying to restrain it.

If a horse is standing with its head away from you in an enclosure, first try to lure it to turn toward you by talking calmly or shaking grain or feedstuff to get its attention. Always be sure to leave an escape route so that you do not get trapped in the stall with the horse. For a calm horse, you can enter the enclosure while talking to the horse. Approach slowly, letting the horse know you are there. If the horse is standing so that it is safer to approach its off shoulder (right = off) (Fig. 6-2, *C* and *D*), slip the lead over its neck and turn the horse so you can apply the halter from its near side (near = left).

Some horses quickly learn that a rope or halter slung over a human's shoulder means they must go to work, and these horses will not allow you to catch them. For these horses, it is best to keep the ropes hidden from view until you are up close. Baling twine or a small rope works well with these horses because it is more easily concealed and need not be very strong; once the horse is caught, it usually submits quietly. More nervous horses must be enclosed in a smaller pen to catch them. Luring them into the pen with grain is much better than chasing them in because they are then less agitated.

If all else fails, try to rope the horse. Again, it is better to have the horse in a fairly small pen for this. Keep your movements slow and deliberate. Do not swing the rope around your head like you are going to rope a calf. It is best to use a low, backhand technique. Hold the rope at waist height and make a large loop that just brushes the ground. The major portion of the rope should be coiled and held loosely in your left hand so it can peel off after you catch the horse. Hold the loop in your right hand on the left side of your body, palm facing toward you, then situate yourself 8 to 10 feet from the fence on your right side.

FIG. 6-2

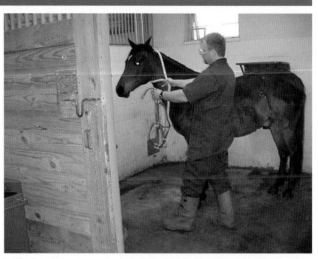

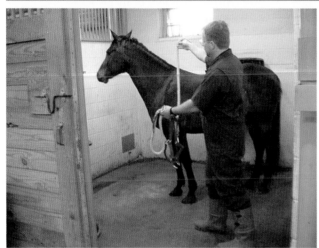

A Horses are trained to be saddled and mounted from the near side.

B Slip the lead rope over the horse's neck and catch the end as it comes into your reach; tie a single overhand knot to keep the rope from slipping off.

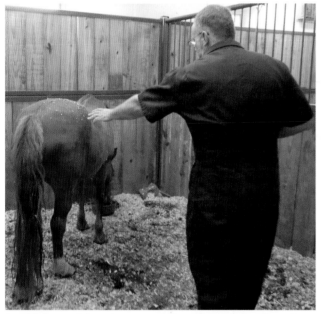

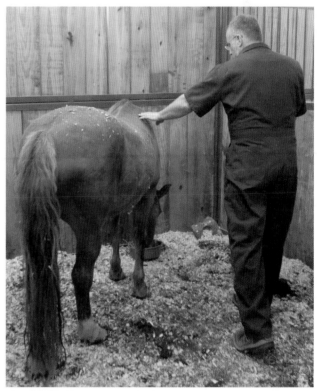

C and D Approach from the rear so the horse knows you are there, then approach to its shoulder to apply the lead rope.

Have another person drive the horse between you and the fence; as it goes by, you can toss the loop up so the horse runs into it. Keeping the horse along the fence prevents it from dodging away from the rope as you toss it, so the person driving the horse between you and the fence must keep it moving. The rope can be snubbed around a post to take up the slack when the horse is caught. Because the roped horse may resist violently, it is wise to wear gloves to protect your hands from rope burns.

The halter and lead rope are the main tools of equine restraint and should always be used when leading or working on a horse. Check the halter and lead rope for splits or fraying, as a horse can easily break a defective lead rope or halter with a sharp jerk of its head.

After you have caught the horse and it has settled down, place the neck strap and the buckle end of the halter in your left hand. Standing on the near side, hold the buckle in your right hand and the neck strap in your left hand, then move up to the horse's muzzle (Fig. 6-3, *A*). Gently slide the noseband around the horse's nose, flip the strap over the poll and on your side of the neck (Fig. 6-3, *B*), and secure the halter by buckling it to the neck strap (Fig. 6-3, *C*). Untie the lead rope from around the horse's neck and find the center ring on the bottom of the halter (Fig. 6-3, *D*). Attach the clip to the center ring (Fig. 6-3, *E*).

FIG. 6-3

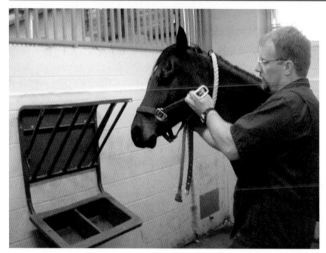

A Standing on the near side, hold the buckle in your right hand and the neck strap in your left hand as you move up to the horse's muzzle.

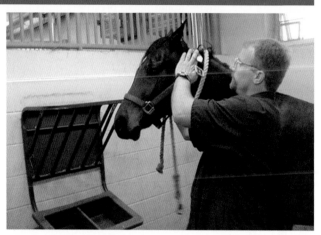

B Gently slide the noseband around the horse's nose and flip the strap over the poll on your side of the neck.

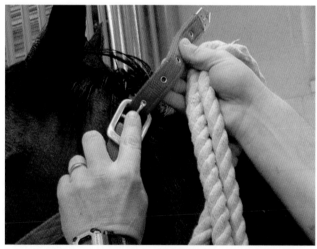

C Secure the halter by buckling it to the neck strap.

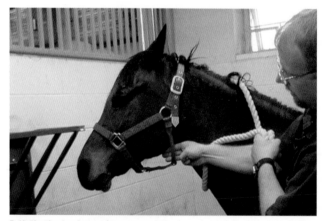

D Untie the lead rope from around the horse's neck and find the center ring on the bottom of the halter.

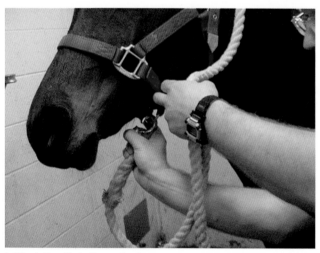

E Attach the clip to the center ring.

Check to make sure the halter is settled correctly on the horse's face. There should be no pressure points from rings or rivets, and the straps should not be close to or over the horse's eyes.

If the horse is "head shy," it may throw its head up or sometimes even rear if a person reaches toward its face. This is usually caused by rough treatment of the horse about its head and neck. To approach this type of horse with the halter, work from the back of its head so the animal does not see the halter approaching. Keep your gestures lower than the muzzle and move slowly and deliberately. Talk to continually reassure the animal.

If you must approach a horse from the rear, as in a box stall or if the animal is tied, always let the horse know you are approaching. Begin to talk quietly to the horse before you get close. Remember that a horse's kicking range is 6 to 8 feet straight back and these kicks are usually very accurate. Talk to the horse before and as you approach it, so you do not surprise or startle it. It is safest to pass behind the horse about 10 to 12 feet or more or to stay in direct physical contact by keeping your hand on the horse's rump when passing around the rear (Fig. 6-4, A and B). This does not guarantee that you will not get kicked; however, if you are kicked, the blow will be reduced and further down on your body, where it is less life threatening.

FIG. 6-4

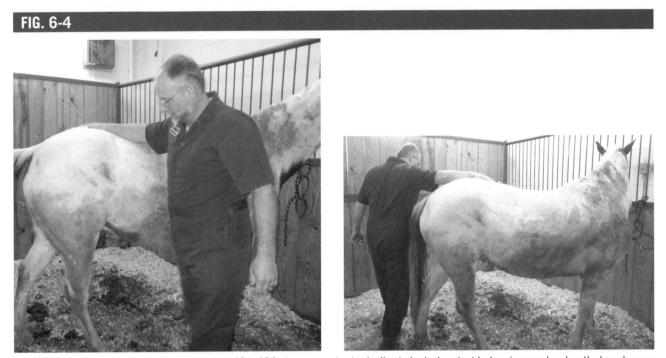

A and B It is safest to pass behind the horse about 10 to 12 feet or more or to stay in direct physical contact by keeping your hand on the horse's rump when passing around the rear.

LEADING A HORSE

Once you have haltered the horse, grasp the lead rope where it connects to the halter with your right hand and use your left hand to hold the loose end of the rope in neat loops, with the entire rope held in front of you (Fig. 6-5, *A* and *B*). Never wrap the loose end of the lead rope around your hand or have the rope running behind you (Fig. 6-5, *C*). If the horse bolts, you will be pulled along with it and could be seriously injured. Always walk on the near side of the horse, close to the shoulder, and hold the lead rope with your right hand about one foot away from the base of the halter (Fig. 6-5, *D*).

After you stop leading a horse, stand as close to its shoulder as possible and face the same direction as the horse. Be careful not to stand too far in front of the horse, as it can rear up and strike with its front foot. Also, do not stand too near or the horse can accidentally step on the back of your heels as you are walking.

Some horses may try to bite you while being led or handled. Deliver punishment at the time of the bite by rapping the horse firmly on its muzzle. You do not usually have to cause pain with such a rap, only convey the impression that you will not tolerate bad behavior. Punishment given too long after the fact is futile.

FIG. 6-5

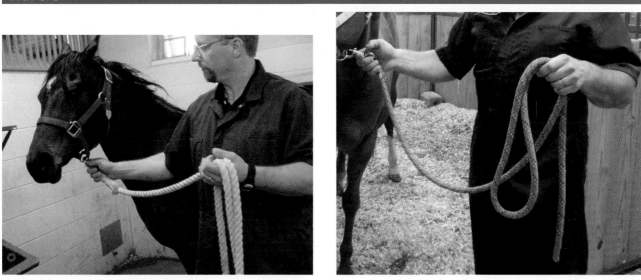

A and B Once the horse is haltered, grasp the lead rope where it connects to the halter with your right hand; your left hand holds the loose end of the rope in neat loops, with the entire rope held in front of you.

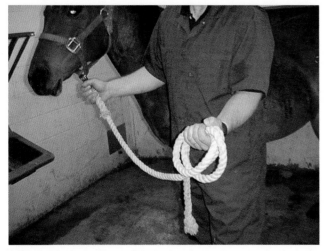

C Never wrap the loose end of the lead rope around your hand or have the rope running behind you.

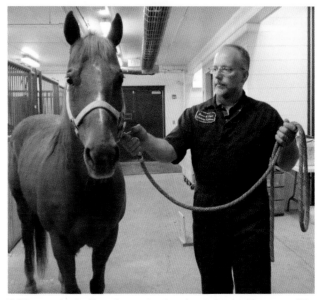

D After you stop leading a horse, stand as close to its shoulder as possible.

TYING A HORSE

The movies would have us believe that a horse will stand quietly in one place until the owner returns, no matter what is going on around it, with only the reins wrapped around a post or dropped to the ground. Unfortunately, this is true only if the horse has been trained to be "ground tied." In most cases, if a horse is to be left unattended, it should always be tied to a sturdy object with a properly fitting halter and suitable lead rope.

The knot used to tie the lead rope should be a quick-release knot, such as the halter tie. Pass the rope around a sturdy post, ideally a vertical post that is placed in the ground (Fig. 6-6, *A*). Allowing 2 to 3 feet of lead for the horse, make a loop that opens up in the end as close to the post as you can and lay it on top of the standing part (Fig. 6-6, *B*). Make a bight in the end; pass it under the standing part and through the loop (Fig. 6-6, *C*). Pull the

bight to tighten the knot (Fig. 6-6, *D*). The quick-release knot allows the horse to be released quickly if it panics, catches its foot, or falls down. To release the knot, simply pull on the end.

The horse should be allowed about 2 to 3 feet of lead rope so it can adjust the angle of its neck and shift position as it desires. Allowing more slack than that may cause the horse to tangle its front feet in the rope. Any less slack may frustrate the horse enough for it to try to escape. Do not tie a horse's head too high or too low so it is at an unnatural angle. Rather, tie it so the horse's head is held in a natural position about level with its withers. Always check the area around a tied horse for possible hazards that could cause serious injuries if the horse were suddenly frightened. Never move under a tied horse's neck to get to the other side. This is very dangerous and could result in injury if the horse is suddenly frightened because it could lunge forward and slam into you.

FIG. 6-6

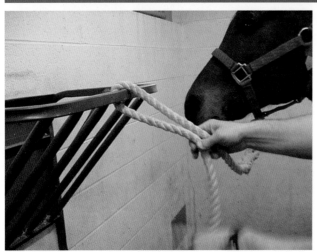

A Pass the rope around a sturdy post, ideally a vertical post that is placed in the ground.

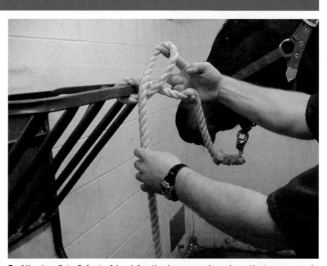

B Allowing 2 to 3 feet of lead for the horse, make a loop that opens up in the end as close to the post as you can and lay it on top of the standing part.

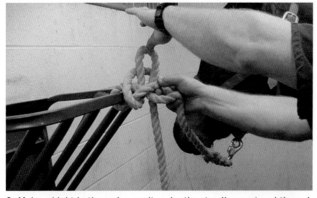

C Make a bight in the end; pass it under the standing part and through the loop.

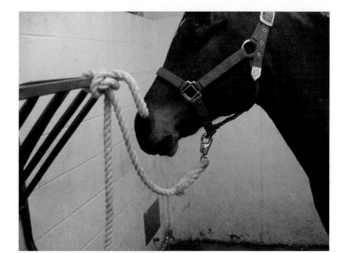

D Pull the bight to tighten the knot.

FIG. 6-7

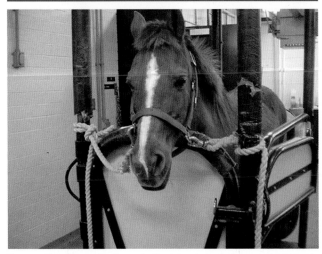

To cross tie, clip one lead rope to the lateral cheek rings on the left side of the horse's halter. Tie the left lead, using the halter tie.

CROSS TYING

Cross tying is another way to secure a horse's head and to keep it from rearing. To cross tie, clip one lead rope to the lateral cheek rings on the left side of the horse's halter. Tie the left lead, using the halter tie. Then walk safely around to the horse's right side and affix the second lead to the lateral cheek ring and tie the horse, again using the halter tie (Fig. 6-7). Do not stand directly in front of the horse. Even with its head secured, the horse can still toss its head or strike out with its front foot.

RESTRAINT OF THE HEAD

For almost every veterinary procedure done on a horse, the head must be restrained. The standard equipment for head restraint is the halter and lead rope. You can use these to hold the horse still, direct its attention elsewhere, and secure it to one spot. Therefore it is important to examine this equipment for worn or broken parts before use. In addition, while using the halter be sure to maintain a firm hold.

You must follow three important rules when restraining a horse. First, always stand on the same side of the horse as the person who is working on the animal. If the horse tries to escape, it usually will move away from you. If there are people on both sides of it, the animal will pick the smaller of the barriers and move over that, possibly resulting in injury to a person bending or kneeling down. You will also have to pay attention to the horse as well as what is going on with the procedure. Too often handlers become so wrapped up in what is going on with the procedure that they miss the signs of the horse getting restless or agitated. Then it is too late to try to calm or

distract the horse or warn the other person to be ready to get out of the way.

The second rule is to keep the horse's head down so that its eye is looking into your eye. If the horse raises its head up above your shoulders, you will not be able to keep it from moving away. To keep the horse's head down, place one hand over the poll, applying a gentle pressure, and pull down on the lead rope. As soon as the horse drops its head stop applying the pressure. This is teaching the horse to keep its head down. The release of the pressure is a reward for doing what you want it to do.

The third rule is to never stand directly in front of a horse. It can rear up and come down on top of you. It can strike out with its front feet or can run you down in an effort to escape. Always stand to the side of the horse, and be prepared for a sudden reaction. Sometimes a halter alone is not adequate restraint, and you must rely on other devices to distract the horse's attention. Distraction techniques can help, but if distraction is not enough, a twitch or a chain or rope shank may be necessary.

DISTRACTION TECHNIQUES

Distraction techniques work well on horses and should be employed as needed. They will keep the horse concentrating on what you are doing versus what the veterinarian may be doing.

Rocking an Ear

Stand on the side of the horse that is being worked on, hold the halter with one hand, and with the other hand grasp the horse's ear at the base and gently rock it or bend it back and forth (Fig. 6-8, *A*). Do not do this too vigorously as you can damage the cartilage and cause the horse's ear to droop. You may also wish to ask the owner if it is okay to use this technique. Show horses often are trimmed up around the ears; if this distraction technique makes them resist having their ears handled, the owner will not be happy.

Skin Roll

Hold the halter in one hand and with the other grasp as much skin on the shoulder as you can get. Rocking it back and forth or jiggling it provides enough distraction to allow you or another person to accomplish intravenous and intramuscular injections (Fig. 6-8, *B*).

Hand Twitch

Hold the halter in one hand so that you have good head control. Grasp or massage the upper lip with your other hand rocking the muzzle back and forth. Be careful not to close off the horse's nostrils (Fig. 6-8*C*). Some horses tire of this or do not like it at all and will fuss so watch and stop this technique if the horse becomes agitated.

FIG. 6-8

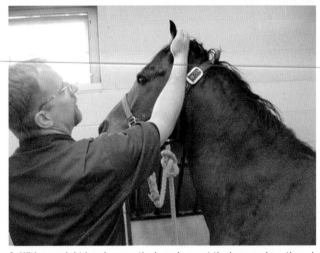

A With your right hand, grasp the horse's ear at the base and gently rock it or bend it back and forth.

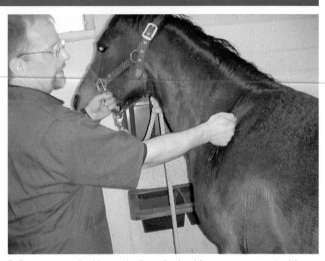

B Grasp as much skin on the horse's shoulder as you can get with one or both hands.

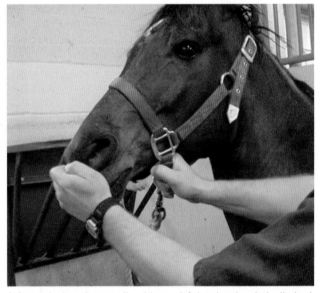

C Grasp the horse's upper lip with your left hand and rock the lip back and forth. Be careful not to close off the horse's nostrils.

Eye Cover

Hold the halter in one hand then slide your other hand up from the cheek and gently cover one eye. You can rock your hand gently or just cup the eye. Do not plop your hand over the eye when first applying this technique. It will startle the horse, and it may try to bolt (Fig. 6-9, *A*).

Blindfolds

If a horse is afraid to enter a trailer, stock rack, or box stall, or is simply obstinate, using a towel as a blindfold may help. The blindfolded horse usually calms down and then depends on you to guide it. Work slowly and talk constantly to reassure the blindfolded horse (Fig. 6-9, *B* and C).

"Caveman Pats"

A flat-handed, firm pat on the cheek, neck, or other area does a great job of distracting a horse from things going on elsewhere. To ensure the horse does not anticipate what will happen, vary the frequency, intensity, and location of pats.

FIG. 6-9

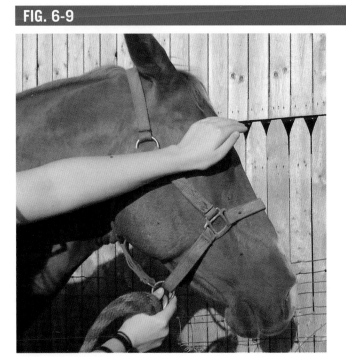

A Slowly cup your hand over the horses' eye.

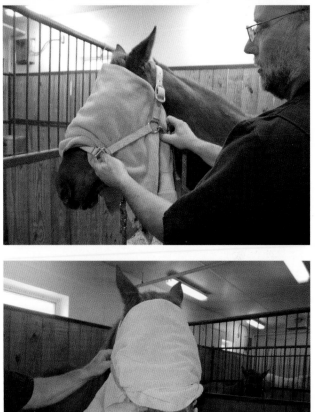

B and C A blindfold over the eyes calms the horse.

Leg Lift

The last technique is quite useful when trying to take a radiograph of a leg. If the horse moves or is unwilling to stand still, lift and hold the leg opposite of the one being radiographed. This will often make the horse stand still. With all techniques, remember the distraction must be intermittent otherwise the horse grows accustom to the distraction and will revert its attention back to the procedure (Fig. 6-10).

FIG. 6-10

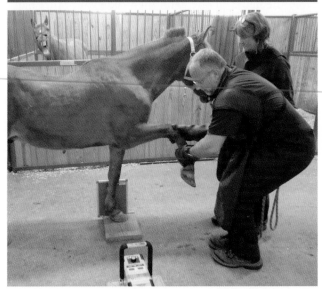

Lifting a leg to force a horse to stand still for a radiograph.

TWITCHES

Common types of twitches used on horses are the chain, humane (or clamp), and rope twitches. All have advantages and disadvantages. Often a client's attitude about twitches dictates which one, if any, is used in a particular situation. Twitches should only be used if you know how to apply them and are often a last resort.

Twitches work only for a short time before the muzzle loses feeling, so the greatest effect is when it is first applied. To maximize the twitch's usefulness, tightening and loosening the loop around the muzzle keeps the circulation flowing and keeps the horse's attention on the twitch longer. Be aware that many horses try to get away or resist the twitch when it is first applied; stay with them by moving with their motions. If they shake you off the first time, it becomes more difficult to place the twitch on again. However, if a horse continues to struggle or escalates the struggle, try another distraction technique or possibly chemical restraint.

After the twitch is removed, massage the muzzle to restore circulation. This also lets the horse know that a person can touch its muzzle without hurting it.

The twitch can be applied to the lower lip of a horse as well but should only be used if the horse raises strong objections to using the upper lip. Always curl the lip inward to protect the inner surface.

The chain twitch is a flat chain loop attached to the end of a stout wooden handle to form a loop. To apply the twitch, hold onto the halter and the twitch handle with your right hand place the loop of chain over your left hand. Catch one side of the loop between your little finger and ring finger to prevent it from slipping down onto your wrist (Fig. 6-11, *A*). Grasp as much of the horse's upper lip with your left hand as possible, pressing the bottom edges together to protect the delicate inner surface (Fig. 6-11, *B*) and quickly slide the handle up so the chain loop rests high up around the lip (Fig. 6-11, *C*). Tighten the chain around the upper lip by twisting the handle (clockwise if on the left side of the head and counterclockwise if on the right) before letting go of the muzzle (Fig. 6-11, *D*). Hold the twitch in your left hand and the halter with your right (Fig. 6-11, *E*).

FIG. 6-11

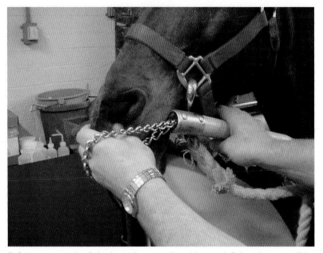

A Catch one side of the loop between your little finger and ring finger to prevent it from slipping down onto your wrist.

B Grasp as much of the horse's upper lip with your left hand as possible, pressing the bottom edges together to protect the delicate inner surface.

(**Figure 6-11,** continued on following page)

FIG. 6-11 cont.

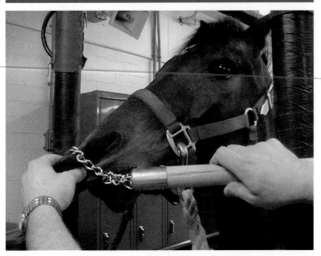

C Quickly slide the handle up so the chain loop rests high up around the horse's lip.

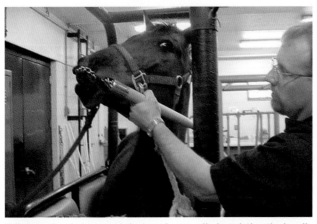

D Tighten the chain around the horse's upper lip by twisting the handle (clockwise if on the left side of the horse's head and counterclockwise if on the right) before letting go of the muzzle.

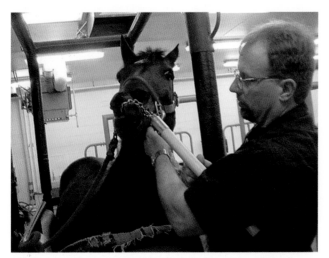

E Hold the twitch in your left hand and the halter with your right.

An advantage of a chain twitch is that it slips off easily when the chain is loosened. The length of the handle is usually long enough for the restrainer to stand back beside the horse and hang onto the halter as well. The chain can be loosened and tightened or gently wiggled for added distraction. If steady pressure is constantly applied, the muzzle loses circulation and becomes numb, rendering the twitch ineffective. A disadvantage is that sometimes the horse learns to wiggle its upper lip to dislodge the twitch (Fig. 6-12). Another disadvantage occurs if the horse pulls the handle out of the handler's hands. The free handle can then become a dangerous weapon if the horse throws its head.

FIG. 6-12

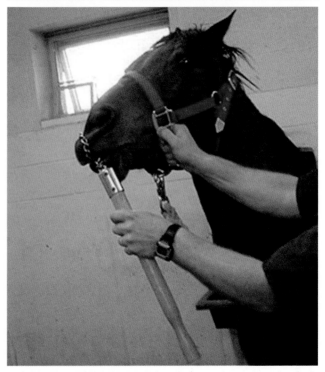

A disadvantage of the chain twitch is that some horses learn to wiggle their upper lip to dislodge it.

The humane twitch is a metal clamp-like device that pinches the upper lip between two bars. The twitch usually has a length of cord with a clasp attached to it that can be wrapped around the end of the twitch and then attached to the halter. Regardless of its name, this twitch is not any more humane or inhumane than the chain or rope twitch.

The primary disadvantage of this twitch is that it applies steady pressure that can cause the lip to lose feeling, thus losing its effectiveness. Also, the twitch can be dislodged and become a hazardous flying object if it is attached to the halter. This can scare the horse, causing it to fight to get away from this strange object. Unfortunately it cannot get away if the twitch is attached to its halter. For this reason, we strongly recommend not clipping the twitch to the halter.

To apply the humane twitch, start by reaching your left hand through the handles (Fig. 6-13, *A*). Grasp the horse's upper lip to roll the lips in before placing the twitch around the muzzle (Fig. 6-13, *B*). Close the twitch by bringing the handles together firmly (Fig. 6-13, *C*). Hold the twitch with your left hand and the halter with your right. Do not twist the muzzle while it is in the twitch, as this causes more pain than is necessary. Simply squeeze or jiggle the muzzle to achieve the desired effect (Fig. 6-13, *D*). The humane twitch will lose its effectiveness in 10 to 20 minutes because the muzzle will lose circulation and go numb.

A rope twitch is made from small-diameter cord attached to a stout handle or ring. It is applied to the horse's muzzle in the same manner as the chain twitch. The advantage of a rope twitch is that it is relatively inexpensive and easily made. Also, the loop tends to stay on the horse's muzzle better than a chain. The disadvantage of the rope muzzle is that it tends to pinch the horse's muzzle more than the chain, often causing unnecessary pain.

FIG. 6-13

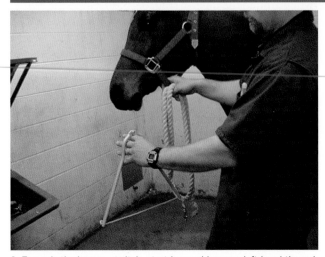

A To apply the humane twitch, start by reaching your left hand through the handles.

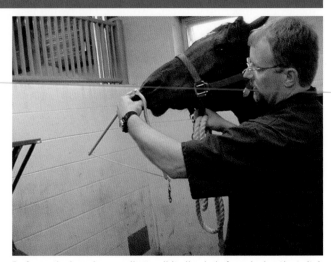

B Grasp the horse's upper lip to roll its lips in before placing the twitch around the muzzle.

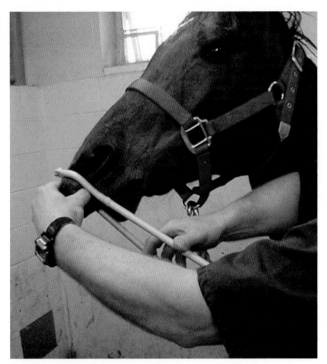

C Close the twitch by bringing the handles together firmly.

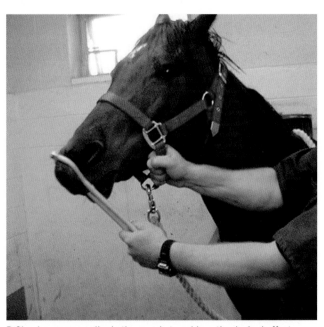

D Simply squeeze or jiggle the muzzle to achieve the desired effect.

CHAIN SHANK

The chain shank (also called a stud shank) is a long leather or nylon strap with about 2 feet of flat chain at its end, attached to a snap. It can be used as another distraction device or on horses that need more restraint than just a halter, such as many stallions. You can use a chain shank in a number of ways.

The first method is the most common. With the halter in place, pass the chain end through the ring on the cheek piece of the near side (Fig. 6-14, *A*) bringing it across the bridge of the horse's nose to the ring on the off side of the head (Fig. 6-14, *B*). The chain is held in the same hand that holds the lead rope. When the horse tosses its head or rears up, you can snap the chain to make the horse stop or pay attention (Fig. 6-14, *C*).

Another way to use the chain shank is to attach the chain as previously described but, instead of leaving it across the bridge of the horse's nose, pass it under the horse's top lip (Fig. 6-14, *D*). This really gets the horse's attention when you snap the chain. Please use it sparingly and only when a horse is being extraordinarily naughty (Fig. 6-14, *E*).

You can also put the chain shank under a horse's chin. This is not recommended, however, as it can cause the horse to throw its head up when the chain is snapped instead of keeping its head down where you can maintain control.

A simpler version of the chain shank is a small diameter piece of nylon rope with a clip on one end. The clip is attached to the side ring on the halter, then the rope is placed under the bottom lip and then threaded through the opposite side ring on the halter. The person restraining the horse then holds onto the rope and if the horse acts up a quick jerk on the rope will call its attention back to the rope. This works great for farrier work because it distracts the horse and does not cause any pain.

FIG. 6-14

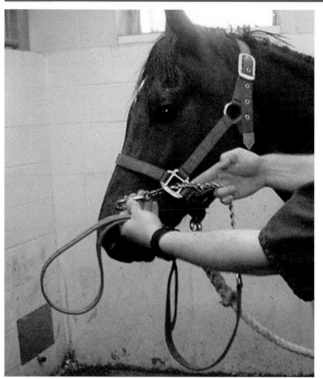

A With the halter in place, pass the chain end through the ring on the cheek piece of the near side.

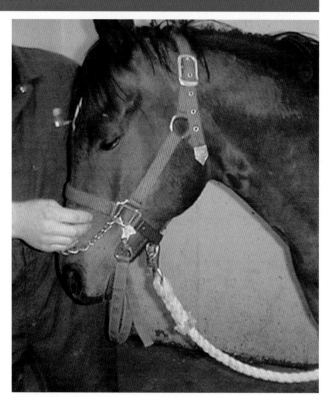

B Next, pass it across the bridge of the horse's nose to the ring on the off side of the horse's head.

(**Figure 6-14,** continued on following page)

FIG. 6-14 cont.

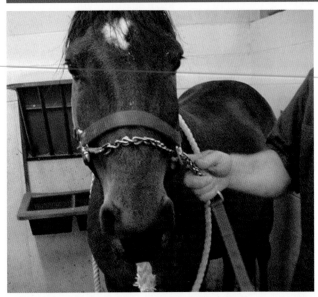

C Hold the chain in the same hand that holds the lead rope.

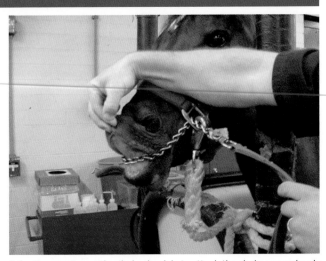

D Another way to use the chain shank is to attach the chain as previously described, but instead of leaving it across the bridge of the horse's nose, pass it under the horse's top lip.

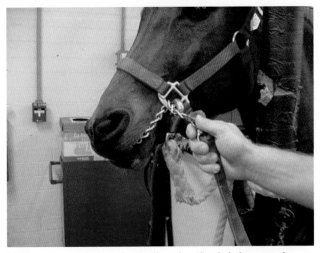

E This really gets the horse's attention when the chain is snapped.

LIFTING FEET

Stand facing the back of the horse, run your hand down the horse's near front leg, and ask it to pick up its foot or say, "Give me your foot" (Fig. 6-15, *A*). As the horse allows you to pick up its foot, be sure to hold the hoof and not the fetlock or pastern because that puts pressure on the joint, which is uncomfortable for the horse.

When the horse has lifted its foot, balance the hoof on your knee (Fig. 6-15, *B*). To clean the hooves, you do not have to put the horse's leg between your knees; farriers will often do this to trim and file hooves. To clean, hold the hoof with your left hand and the hoof pick with your right hand (Fig. 6-15, *C*). Move the pick from the heel to the toe in a motion away from the body (Fig. 6-15, *D*).

FIG. 6-15

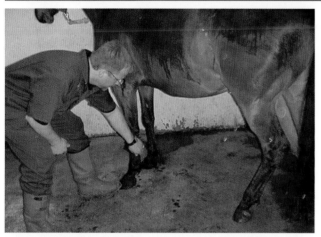

A Stand facing the back of the horse, and run your hand down the horse's near front leg; ask the horse to pick its foot up or say, "Give me your foot."

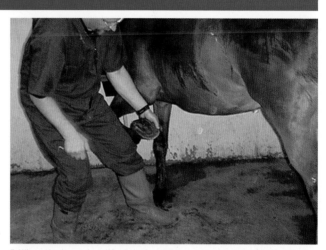

B When the horse has lifted its foot, balance the hoof on your knee.

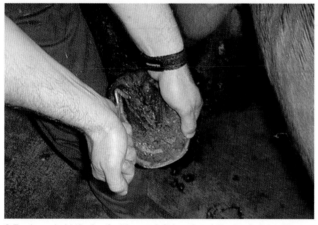

C To clean, hold the hoof with your left hand and the hoof pick with your right hand.

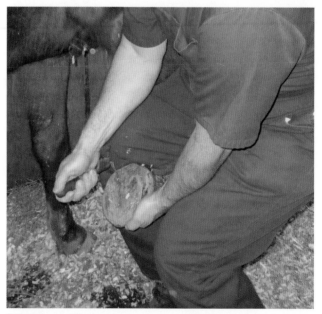

D Hold the hoof firmly between your legs so that you do not cause movement of the pastern joint.

To lift the rear foot, stand facing the back of the horse, fairly close to the side of its hindquarters. Run your hand down the horse's near leg and ask it to give you its foot as you get to just above the pastern (Fig. 6-16, *A*). As the horse gives you its foot, move forward a bit to stretch its leg out while you place its hoof on your thigh (Fig. 6-16, *B*). If the horse starts to pull the foot away, grasp it with both hands to steady it on your knee (Fig. 6-16, *C*). To clean the hoof out, move the pick from the heel to the toe.

FIG. 6-16

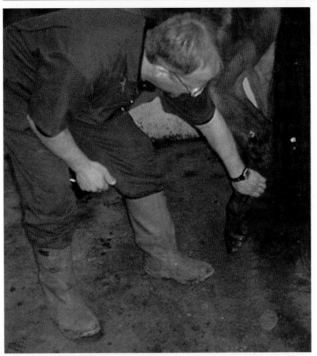

A Run your hand down the horse's near leg and ask it to give you its foot as you get to just above the pastern.

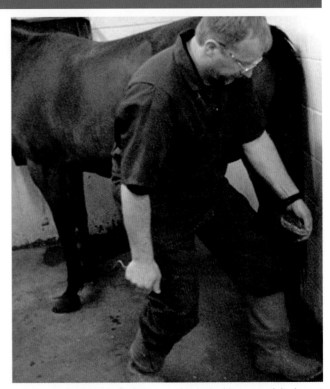

B As the horse gives you its foot, move forward a bit to stretch its leg out while you place the hoof on your thigh.

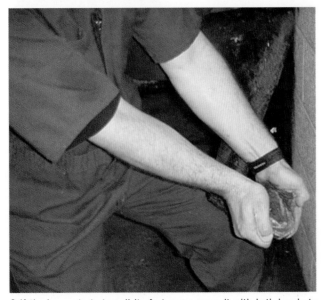

C If the horse starts to pull its foot away, grasp it with both hands to steady it on your knee.

PLACING A MOUTH WEDGE

Hold the mouth wedge in your left hand and the halter at the cheek band with your right hand (Fig. 6-17, *A*) Reach your right thumb into the corner of the horse's mouth and insert the wedge in as the horse opens its mouth from the pressure of your thumb (Fig. 6-17, *B*). Start the mouth wedge into the horse's mouth until it is seated between the horse's jaws and molars (Fig. 6-17, *C*).

FIG. 6-17

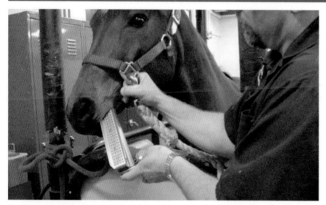

A Hold the mouth wedge in your left hand and the halter at the cheek band with your right hand.

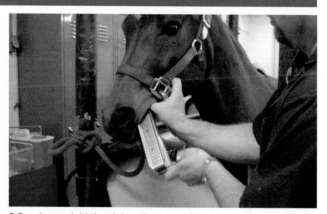

B Reach your right thumb into the corner of the horse's mouth and insert the wedge as the horse opens its mouth from the pressure of your thumb.

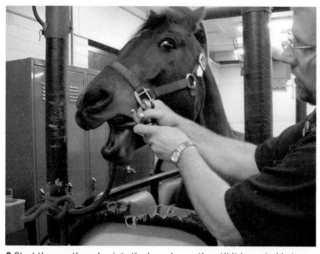

C Start the mouth wedge into the horse's mouth until it is seated between the horse's jaws and molars.

STOCKS

Stocks are narrow enclosures with removable or semiopen sides and a gate at both ends. They can be made of steel pipes or wooden planks, with the top bar or plank no higher than the horse's shoulder. The front of the stocks should have the necessary hooks for cross tying so the horse cannot jump forward or to the side if it tries to escape. A gate is included at both ends because horses do not like narrow, confined areas. The opened front gate gives the appearance of an escape route as the horse is walked into the stocks (see Fig. 6-18, *A*, for a rear view of the stocks).

After opening both gates, lead the horse up to the back gate and step to the outside of the stocks. Do not go into the stocks. Pass the rope around the bars as needed to keep the horse moving. Have someone gently close the front and back gates as soon as the horse is properly situated inside. A horse should not be left unattended when placed in the stocks (Fig. 6-18, *B*).

FIG. 6-18

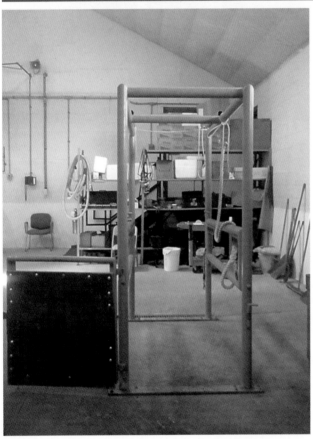

A This is a picture of what the horse sees as it enters the stocks.

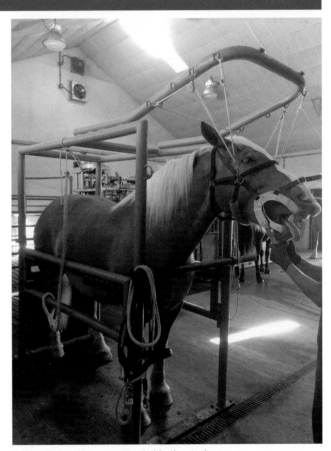

B Never leave a horse unattended in the stocks.

TAIL TYING

Much of a horse's weight can be raised or moved by its tail, which is quite strong. This makes the tail a handy object to use when you need to move an anesthetized horse. However, the tail can also be a nuisance that must be tied out of the way for certain procedures. Remember to always tie the tail to the animal's own body, as severe injury may result if the tail is tied to an immovable object and the horse suddenly bolts.

To secure a cord or rope to the tail, first find the last coccygeal vertebra of the tail. Gather the hair up and make a bight with the hair so that the vertebra is on one side and the gathered hair is on the other side of the bight. Support the tail in your hand while you bring the end of the rope through the bight (Fig. 6-19, *A*). Pass the end of the rope around the bight so it ends up on top. Bring the end under the rope that is looped around the tail (Fig. 6-19, *B*). Tighten by pulling the short end and the long end together (Fig. 6-19, *C*). You can now tie the long portion of the rope to one of the horse's front legs or its neck using a bowline knot (Fig. 6-19, *D*).

FIG. 6-19

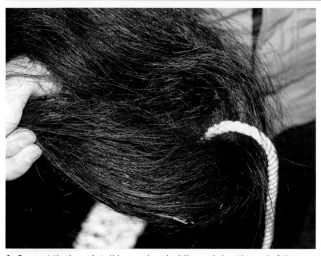

A Support the horse's tail in your hand while you bring the end of the rope through the bight.

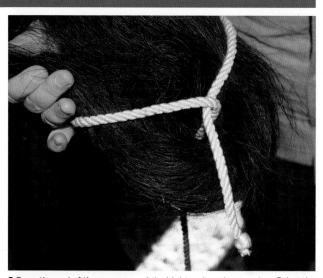

B Pass the end of the rope around the bight so it ends up on top. Bring the end under it until it is looped around the horse's tail.

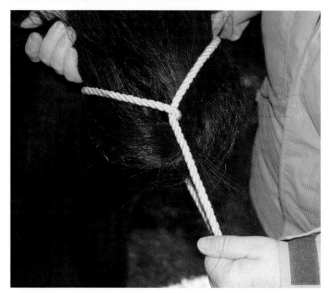

C Tighten by pulling the short end and the long end together.

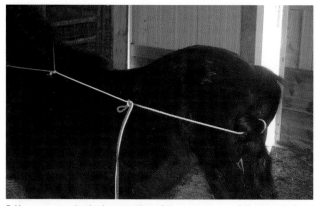

D You can now tie the long portion of the rope to one of the horse's front legs or the neck using a bowline knot.

HOBBLES

Breeding hobbles are used to prevent obstinate mares from kicking the stallion when mounting. These hobbles can also be used for rectal or vaginal palpation if stocks are unavailable. Start with a long rope with a bowline on a bight tied in the center. Place the loop around the horse's neck and tie the long ends to each leg above the hock with a halter tie or clove hitch. Place a couple of bales of straw or hay behind the horse for added security just in case the horse can still move its back legs.

RESTRAINT OF FOALS

The easiest way to catch a foal is to back the mare into the corner of a large box stall and secure her in place. The foal naturally tries to hide behind the mare's flank. When it begins to move, grasp the foal around the front of its chest with one arm and quickly around the rump or grasp its tail with your other hand. Once you have stopped the foal's forward motion, it will typically try to escape by moving backward.

After you have caught the foal, press it up against the wall or a sturdy partition. If this is not feasible, have another person hold the foal in the same manner on the opposite side. Before capturing the foal, make sure the wall or partition does not have holes through which the foal might put its legs, which could cause injuries.

Do not hold onto the foal's tail too tightly or press it down between the legs, as this sometimes makes the foal sit down. Also, never lift a foal off its feet. This makes foals very nervous and they struggle fiercely to regain their feet.

Always talk to and comfort a foal when handling it. Rough handling leads to behavior problems later in life.

Finally, never remove a foal from the sight of the mare. Both mare and foal will fret until they are reunited and both may injure themselves trying to get back together. Securely tying the dam and keeping the foal within the mare's sight can prevent such problems.

LOADING INTO A TRAILER

Horses have long-term memories. It is important that they learn new skills correctly the first time. Unfortunately many have learned trailering can be a trying, fearful experience (for the horse and the hauler).

Be sure the trailer is well lit and provides good level footing (Fig. 6-20, *A*). Allow the horse to see where you want it to go (Fig. 6-20, *B*). Approach the trailer leading the horse as you would lead it into any other situation, looking where you want to go. Hold the lead loosely in your hand so it can slide through your fingers, so that if the horse balks it will not pull you over (Fig. 6-20, *C*). Remember to always have a safe exit route planned so that you do not get pinned in the trailer (Fig. 6-20, *D*). Confidently walk the horse into the trailer and tie it off with a quick release knot or safety clip.

To remove a horse from the trailer it should be backed slowly to the edge of the trailer, allowing it to step off. This is the safest way to unload a horse (Fig. 6-20, *E to G*). Some will allow a horse to turn and walk out of the trailer

FIG. 6-20

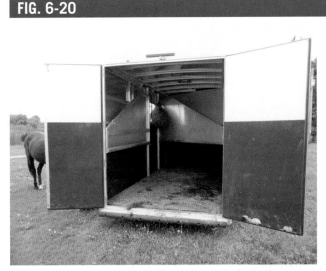

A Be sure the interior of the trailer is well lit and the footing is secure.

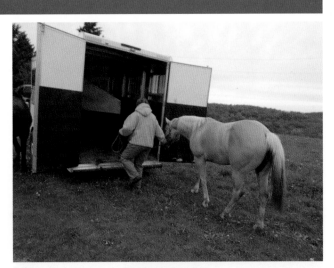

B Allow the horse to see where you expect it to go.

(**Figure 6-20,** continued on following page)

FIG. 6-20 cont.

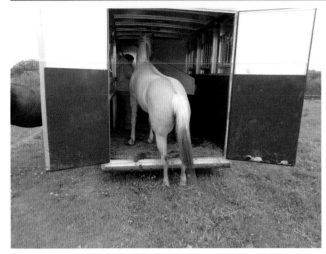

C Confidently lead the horse into the trailer.

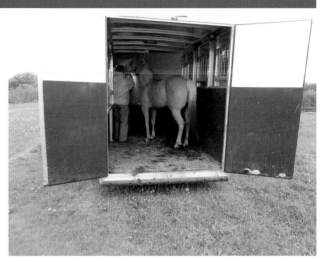

D Ensure you do not get pinned in the trailer and have an exit route planned.

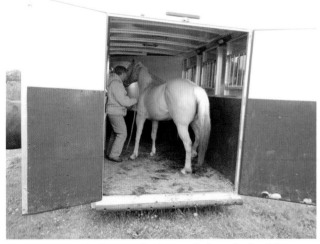

E If possible, turn the horse so that it can exit the trailer head first.

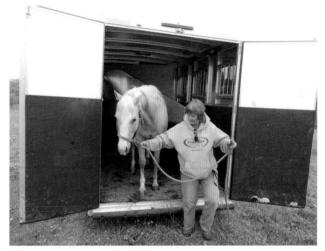

F Allow the horse to slowly exit the trailer.

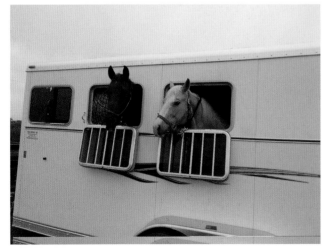

G Happy trails to you!

face first; however, you must be very careful the horse doesn't bolt and drag you off the trailer and not to get too far in front of the horse, as it may come down on top of you if you should falter or go too slow.

If the horse balks at going into the trailer several techniques can be tried. The first is to lunge the horse next to the trailer for a few minutes. When you ask it to stop, move it quickly toward the trailer door and walk up with it into the trailer. If it should balk again, repeat! The horse will soon learn, "If I don't go into the trailer I have to run!"

SUGGESTED READINGS

Blanchard S: Here's how to read your horse's body language, *Pet Health News*, May 25, 1984.

Fowler ME: *Restraint and handling of wild and domestic animals*, Ames, IA, 1978, Iowa State University Press.

Leahy JR, Barrow P: *Restraint of animals*, Ithaca, NY, 1953, Cornell Campus Store.

Nelson B: Restraining horses, *Western Horseman*: 89–94, October 1980.

Roberts M: *Horse sense for people*, New York, 2002, Penguin Books.

Sonsthagen TF: *Restraint of domestic animals*, St. Louis, 1991, Mosby.

Strickland C: How to tie your horse safely and securely, *Horse Illustrated* 39–43, May 1988.

Todd-Jenkins K, Dugan B, Remsburg DW, Montgomery C: Restraint and handling of animals. In *McCurnin's clinical textbook for veterinary technicians*, ed 8, Philadelphia, PA, 2014, Saunders.

Vail C: Tips on equine dentistry, *Norden News*: 15–17, Summer 1980.

Vaughan JT, Allen R: Restraint of horses: part I—head restraint, *Mod Vet Pract* 68:373–383, 1987.

7

Restraint of Sheep

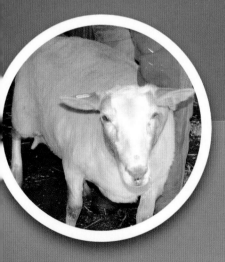
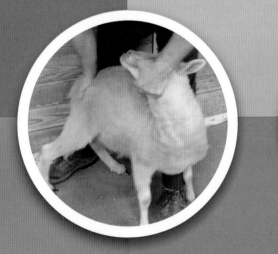
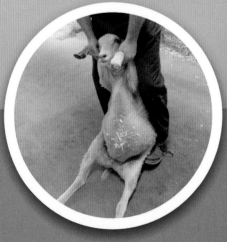

Sheep are easy creatures to restrain if you consider their intense instinct to remain with the flock. This is their main means of defense. By moving as a flock, each member has a better chance of escaping danger. If one sheep requires treatment, the flock experiences less stress if it is allowed to move into a small pen together and the individual needing treatment is then removed.

Sheep show they are disturbed by stamping their front feet or butting with their heads. Rams are especially fond of butting and do so with little provocation, particularly during breeding season. Ewes will also butt especially if they have a lamb to protect. This, along with movement as a group and their speed, is their only means of defense.

Always work with assurance around sheep. Stay calm and be gentle. Sheep can be severely injured by improper restraint. They have fragile bones that can be easily broken by a careless handler. Be aware of this when you grasp a body part.

Sheep with a full coat of wool can become hyperthermic if they are chased and if the weather is warm. If the wool is pulled out in a struggle, the value of the fleece is reduced. Even if the fleece is not pulled out but just pulled on, a subcutaneous bruise can reduce the carcass value and cause pain.

CAPTURING SHEEP

The easiest way to separate an individual from the flock is to drive the entire flock into a small pen or enclosure. Approach the individual slowly. When you are close, swing your arm around the animal's neck and front quarters and quickly wrap your other arm around its rear quarters, grasping the dock (Fig. 7-1). This method of restraint allows you to steer the animal into another pen or move it to a treatment area.

You can also use a shepherd's crook to capture a sheep by hooking a back leg in the area of the hock. Hook and immobilize the animal quickly so it does not have an opportunity to fight the crook and possibly break a leg. Do not use the crook around the animal's neck or more distally on the leg because it can cause severe damage.

Halters can be used on sheep; however, they have short noses and you must be careful that the noseband does not slip down and occlude the animal's nostrils.

RESTRAINT FOR EXAMINATION

If you plan to examine the dorsal aspect of the animal's body, trim its hooves, shear its wool, or give it a subcutaneous vaccination, the easiest method of restraint is to set the animal up on its rump. Most sheep do not seem to object strongly to this technique and are relatively easy to tip onto their rumps. One method is to stand on the left side of the animal with its body parallel to your legs. Place your left knee against the animal's shoulder. Use your hand to check the forward motion of the sheep, with

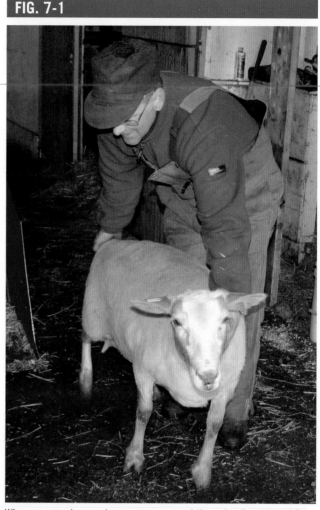

FIG. 7-1

When you are close, swing your arm around the animal's neck and front quarters, and quickly wrap your other arm around its rear quarters, grasping the dock.

one hand on the animal's chin and the other on the dock (Fig. 7-2, *A*). With your right hand, reach over the back and grasp the flank on the right side of the sheep. Move the sheep's head to the right toward its shoulder (Fig. 7-2, *B*). Simultaneously step back with your right leg, lift the flank up, and throw the sheep off balance (Fig. 7-2, *C*). With a quick twist you can set it up on its rump. Then move behind the sheep so your legs can brace the sheep's back (Fig. 7-2, *D*). Tilt the animal back so it is sitting at about a 60-degree angle to keep it from struggling to right itself (Fig. 7-2, *E*). It also allows you to let go of the animal so your hands are free to trim hooves, give injections, or shear. Be careful of the front legs because some sheep flail them about and could injure your face.

When releasing the sheep, control the animal to the ground. It is important that the sheep not feel that they are falling because they will flail their legs and strike the restrainer. Large sheep and pregnant ewes should always be guided to the ground.

CHAPTER 7

FIG. 7-2

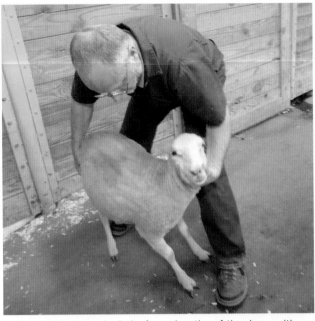

A Use your hands to check the forward motion of the sheep, with one hand on the chin and the other on the dock.

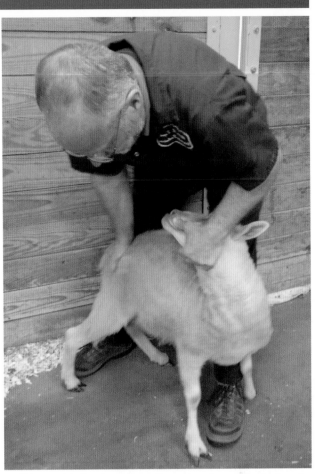

B With your right hand, reach over the back and grasp the flank on the right side of the sheep. Move the sheep's head to the right toward its shoulder.

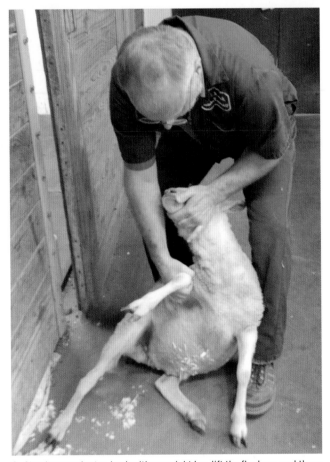

C Simultaneously step back with your right leg, lift the flank up, and throw the sheep off balance. To release the sheep you will gently reverse these steps, turn its head toward its shoulder and gently lower it to the ground.

(**Figure 7-2,** continued on following page)

FIG. 7-2 cont.

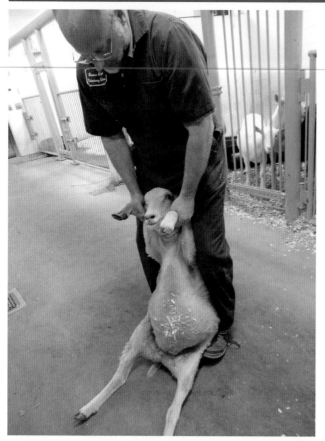

D With a quick twist you can set it up on its rump. Then move behind the sheep so your legs can brace the sheep's back.

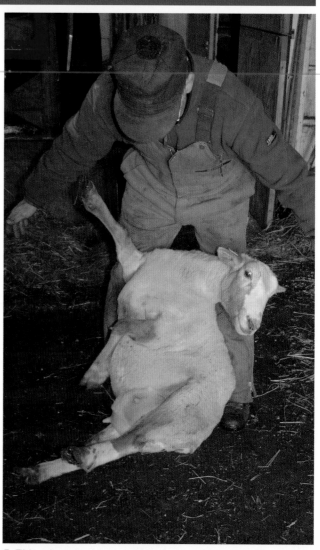

E Tilting the animal back so it is sitting at about a 60-degree angle keeps it from struggling to right itself.

FIG. 7-3

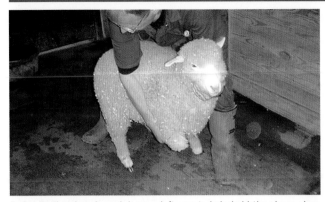

A Cradle the sheep's neck in your left arm to help hold the sheep close to your body. Reach across the sheep and grab its front leg with your right hand.

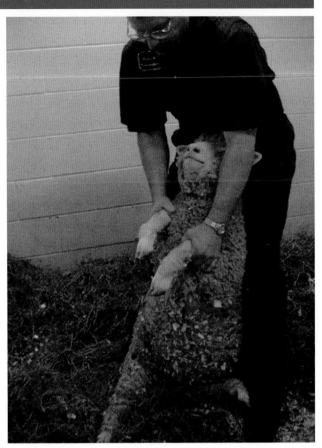

An alternative technique is to place the sheep parallel to your legs. Cradle the neck in your left arm to help hold the sheep close to your body. Reach across the sheep and grab its front leg with your right hand (Fig. 7-3, *A*). Fold the leg up to the animal's body and stand up straight (Fig. 7-3, *B*). This trips the sheep over your right foot. Set the sheep back on its rump as mentioned previously.

B Fold the leg up to the sheep's body and stand up straight.

FIG. 7-4

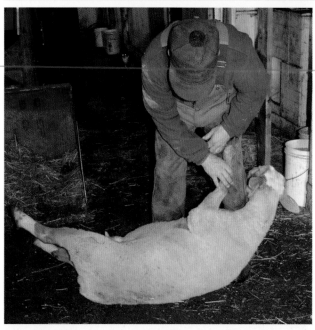

A If you need the sheep to be in lateral recumbency from setting up, you can turn it so the front legs go in between your legs.

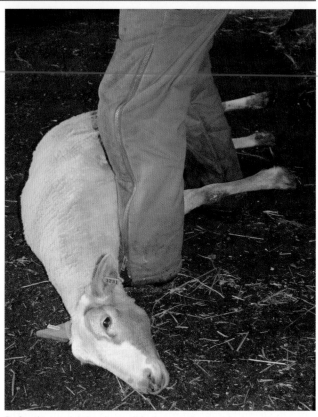

B Continue to let the sheep slide down so its shoulder is resting on your foot.

If you need the sheep to be in lateral recumbency, you can turn it so the front legs go in between your legs (Fig. 7-4, *A*). Continue to let the sheep slide down so its shoulder is resting on your foot (Fig. 7-4, *B*). As long as its shoulder is raised off the ground, the animal will not be able to right itself, allowing you access to the side of the sheep.

If working with young sheep, keep in mind that the tail was likely amputated mere weeks or months earlier and the area may still be sore. If you tuck the animal further back on its rump, it will be more comfortable.

You can give the sheep a physical examination, administer a subcutaneous injection, or trim its feet in this position. This is also the position most shearers use to remove the wool from the sheep.

To return a sheep to its feet, grasp it around the jaw and allow it to rock forward (Fig. 7-5).

FIG. 7-5

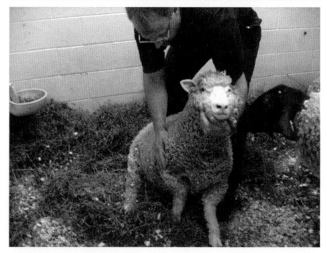

An alternative method of release is to grasp it around the jaw and allow it to rock forward.

RESTRAINT FOR MEDICATIONS

Oral medication for sheep typically is in the form of individual boluses or a drenching solution. To medicate a single sheep in a pen, back the animal into a corner or along a solid wall. Use your knee to pin its neck against the wall, allowing you to reach around its neck and hold its head so that you can administer the medication (Fig. 7-6, *A*). You can also use this technique to hold a sheep in place for intramuscular or subcutaneous injections. If the sheep is small enough or you are tall enough, you can straddle the sheep's neck after backing it into a corner (Fig. 7-6, *B*).

Another method for delivering oral medication is to run a few head of sheep into a squeeze pen or small box stall so that there is little or no room for movement. Then wade in among them. Grasp the animal's jaw to elevate its head so it is nearly perpendicular to the ground and give the medication. Once you have administered the medication, lower the animal's head somewhat to allow it to swallow. Use a marking crayon to mark each sheep after it has been medicated to prevent double dosing.

FIG. 7-6

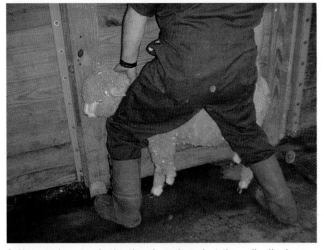

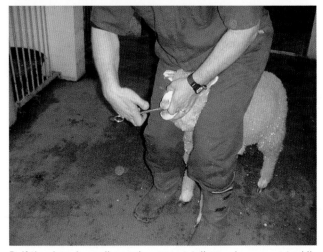

A Use your knee to pin the sheep's neck against the wall, allowing you to reach around its neck and hold its head so that you can give the medication.

B If the sheep is small enough or you are tall enough, you can straddle the sheep's neck after backing it into a corner.

RESTRAINT FOR JUGULAR VENIPUNCTURE

Sheep stocks greatly facilitate restraint for jugular venipuncture. The animal's head is restrained and lateral movements are restricted quite well with the animal in the stocks. However, many farms do not have stocks and it is necessary to manually restrain the sheep for venipuncture.

Start by capturing the sheep in the method described for medicating. Maneuver the sheep around so its rear quarters are in a corner and one side is against the wall. Then straddle the animal, elevate its head, and tuck its head under your arm. You can locate the animal's jugular vein once you part down through the wool to the skin and occlude the vessel in the jugular groove (Fig. 7-7, *A*). If the sheep is too tall to straddle, push the sheep sideways against the wall and stand on the opposite side. Keep the sheep against the wall with your legs and hold its head up as described previously for oral medication.

Jugular venipuncture is also possible with the sheep set up on its rump. Tuck the animal's head below your elbow to restrain it (Fig. 7-7, *B*). This hold can also be used for cephalic venipuncture. The vein sits up on the animal's front leg similarly to that of a dog.

FIG. 7-7

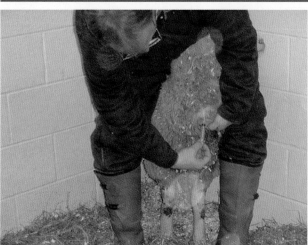

A The jugular vein can be found once you part down through the sheep's wool to the skin and occlude the vessel in the jugular groove.

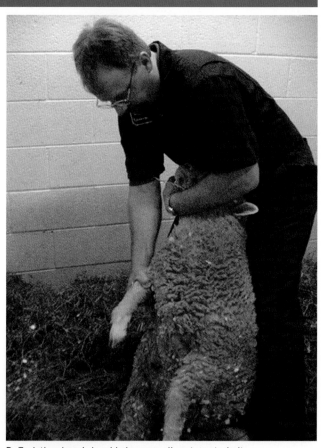

B Tuck the sheep's head below your elbow to restrain it.

FIG. 7-8

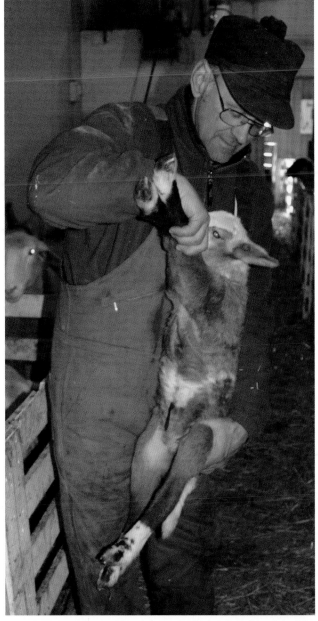

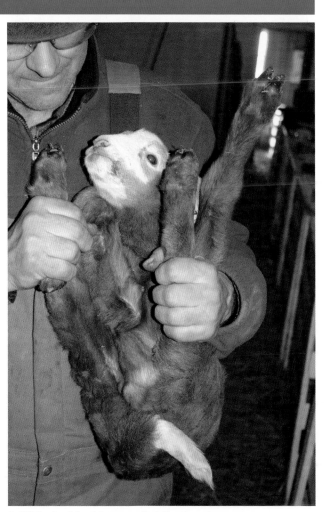

B Tilt the lamb back to expose its tail and scrotum.

A Newborn lambs are easily carried by grasping both front legs with one hand.

RESTRAINT OF LAMBS

You can easily carry newborn lambs by grasping both front legs with one hand (Fig. 7-8, *A*). An alternative method is to place your hand between the lamb's front legs, with its sternum resting on your forearm, much like carrying a small dog. Large lambs are handled as adults.

Restraint for castration and tail docking is relatively easy. The lambs should be placed in a small pen so you do not have to chase them around to capture them. After you have captured one, grasp the front leg and rear leg on the same side in each hand with your right hand grasping the right side and your left hand grasping the left side. Flip the animal so that its back is resting against your chest or lap if you are sitting down. Tilt the lamb back to expose its tail and scrotum (Fig. 7-8, *B*).

SUGGESTED READINGS

Faler K, Faler K: Restraint of sheep, *Mod Vet Pract* 68:562–563, 1987.

Fowler ME: *Restraint and handling of wild and domestic animals*, Ames, IA, 1978, Iowa State University Press.

Leahy JR, Barrow P: *Restraint of animals*, Ithaca, NY, 1953, Cornell Campus Store.

Sonsthagen TF: *Restraint of domestic animals*, St. Louis, 1991, Mosby.

Todd-Jenkins K, Dugan B, Remsburg DW, Montgomery C: Restraint and handling of animals. In *McCurnin's clinical textbook for veterinary technicians*, ed 8, Philadelphia, 2014, Saunders.

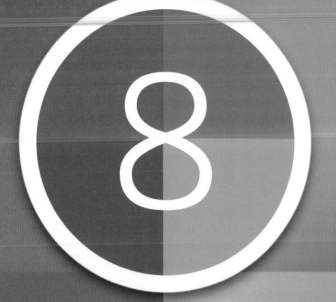

Restraint of Goats

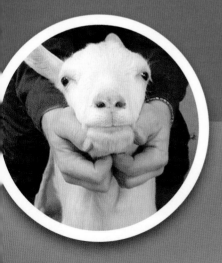

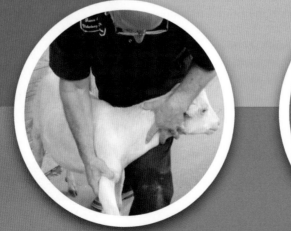

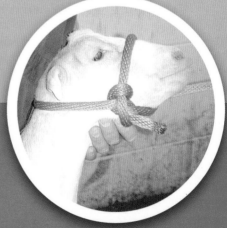

Goats do not tolerate rough treatment and will struggle if improperly handled. For this reason, use the minimum amount of restraint necessary to complete medical procedures on goats.

Contrary to popular belief, goats cannot be treated like sheep. They do not have the same strong instincts to remain with a group as do sheep, and they are more likely to scatter if you try to herd them. It is better to identify the lead goat, usually a doe, and guide her into the barn or pen; the rest of the goats will likely follow.

Goats are usually docile and easily handled. However, you must be friendly or they will become agitated and try to butt you. Signs of impending aggression include holding the tail close to the back with the hair raised along the spine, sneezing, snorting, and stamping. If you ignore these signals, the goat may rear up on its hind legs and butt you.

RESTRAINT FOR EXAMINATION

Use walls or fences to help restrain a goat for short medical procedures. Push the goat's body against the fence or wall with your legs and hips, leaving your hands free for the procedure (Fig. 8-1, *A*). Placing the goat's hindquarters toward a corner is another good technique. Placing your arm around the goat's neck will help keep it still. This works well while completing injections and for determining the animal's temperature, pulse, and respiratory rates (Fig. 8-1, *B* and *C*).

To capture a goat and have it remain still, grasp one of its front legs and lift it (Fig. 8-1, *D*). Most goats stand peacefully when restrained in this way, allowing most types of procedures to be done. This technique works well with both large and small goats. The rear leg can be used for capturing a goat, but it is not a good restraint technique since the goat usually kicks out and struggles. Sometimes, however, grasping the hind leg is the only way to capture a goat. Once you catch the animal, use another restraint technique.

Unlike sheep, goats resent being set up on their rumps. They lash out with their front legs and are usually agile enough to squirm out of the hold. A better method is to lay the goat on its side or flank it.

FIG. 8-1

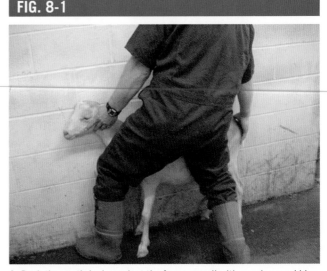

A Push the goat's body against the fence or wall with your legs and hips, leaving your hands free for the procedure.

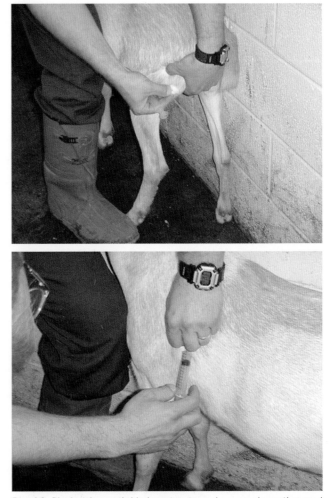

B and C Placing the goat's hindquarters toward a corner is another good technique. Placing your arm around the goat's neck will help keep it still.

(**Figure 8-1,** continued on following page)

FIG. 8-1 cont.

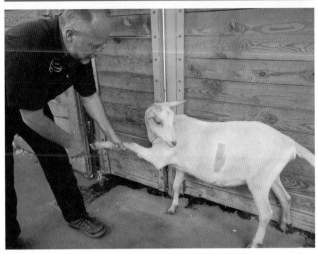

D To capture a goat and have it remain still, grasp one of its front legs and lift it.

There are two methods for flanking a goat. The first positions the goat's body parallel to your legs. Grasp the goat's nose with one hand and its inside (near) rear leg with the other. Bring the goat's leg forward and its nose back to meet the leg. This throws the goat off balance, causing it to fall to the ground.

The second method also positions the goat's body parallel to your legs. Reach over the goat's back and grasp its near front leg while using your forearm to control its head and neck (Fig. 8-2, *A*). Raise its back legs by grasping the flank and lifting (Fig. 8-2, *B*). Gently and carefully put the goat down onto the ground. Once the goat is down, firmly hold all four legs and gently press your knee on the goat's neck to keep the animal recumbent (Fig. 8-2, *C*).

FIG. 8-2

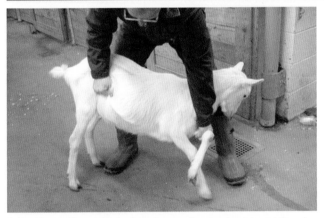

A Reach over the goat's back and grasp its near front leg while using your forearm to control its head and neck.

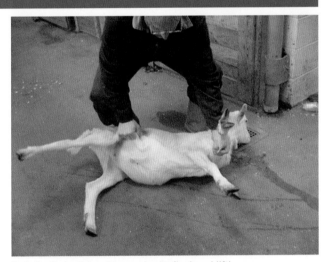

B Raise its back legs by grasping its flank and lifting.

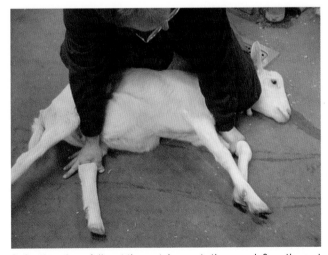

C Gently and carefully put the goat down onto the ground. Once the goat is down, firmly hold all four legs and gently press your knee on the goat's neck to keep the animal recumbent.

RESTRAINT OF THE HEAD

Head restraint is necessary for eye examinations, oral medication administration, or jugular venipuncture. The technique used depends on your preference or the circumstances. Head restraint techniques work best if the goat is backed into a corner and pushed sideways against the wall. This keeps the animal from backing up or moving to the side.

The first technique involves grasping the goat's beard with one hand and encircling its neck with the other hand to stabilize its head (Fig. 8-3). Most goats do not object to this technique, though there is a disadvantage to it. During mating season, male goats urinate on their beards to attract females. This strong odor tends to permeate your clothing and skin.

The second technique is to control the goat's head by placing one hand on either side of its cheeks, wrapping your fingers around its mandible, and holding firmly (Fig. 8-4). This stabilizes the goat's head for jugular venipuncture and eye examination.

Use the goat's horns to capture and lead it for short distances. However, you should switch to a different hold as soon as possible because goats resent having their horns handled and may butt or lash out with their feet.

COLLARS

A neck chain or leather collar is usually used on dairy goats, and they soon become accustomed to being led or restrained by the collar. Collars are useful for securing the goats to a stanchion or wall for such procedures as milking, jugular venipuncture, and general examinations. Collars can be left on the goat permanently. Neck chains should be made of small, flat links that will not catch easily if the goat rubs against a fence. Halters work well on goats, but you have to make sure the noseband does not occlude the goat's nares (Fig. 8-5).

FIG. 8-3

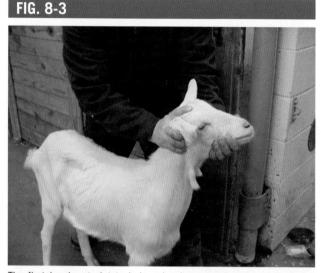

The first head-restraint technique involves grasping the goat's beard with one hand and encircling its neck with your other hand to stabilize its head.

FIG. 8-4

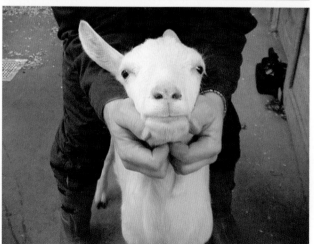

In the second head-restraint method, control the head by placing one hand on either side of the goat's cheeks, wrapping your fingers around its mandible, and holding firmly.

FIG. 8-5

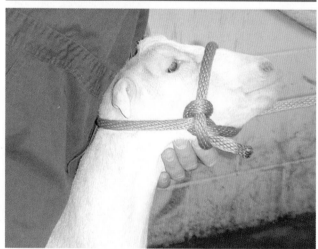

Halters work well on goats, but you have to make sure the noseband does not occlude the nares.

RESTRAINT FOR VENIPUNCTURE

The cephalic veins of goats are much like those of dogs, and the restraint technique used is similar to that used for dogs. Place one hand around the goat's neck to stabilize its head and body and use the other hand to grasp the front leg to be used. Wrap your thumb across the top of the goat's leg and roll the vein out to the top of the leg (Fig. 8-6, *A* and *B*). The person completing the venipuncture must hold the distal portion of the goat's leg while withdrawing the blood sample.

FIG. 8-6

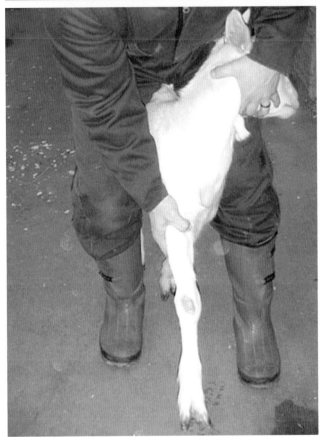

A Straddle the goat and wrap your thumb across the top of the goat's leg and roll the vein out to the top of the leg.

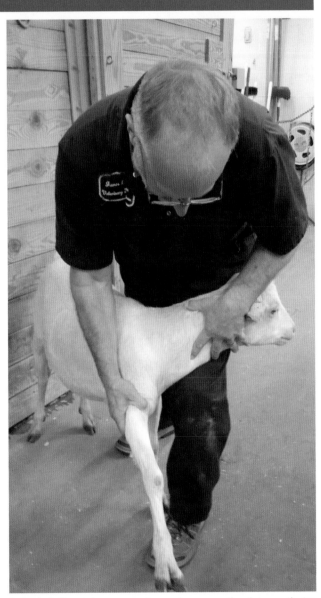

B Restrain the goat across your legs and wrap your thumb across the top of the goat's leg and roll the vein out to the top of the leg.

For jugular venipuncture, back the goat into a corner and push it sideways against the wall. Use one hand to hold the goat's head to the side, and use the other hand to occlude the vessel (Fig. 8-7).

FIG. 8-7

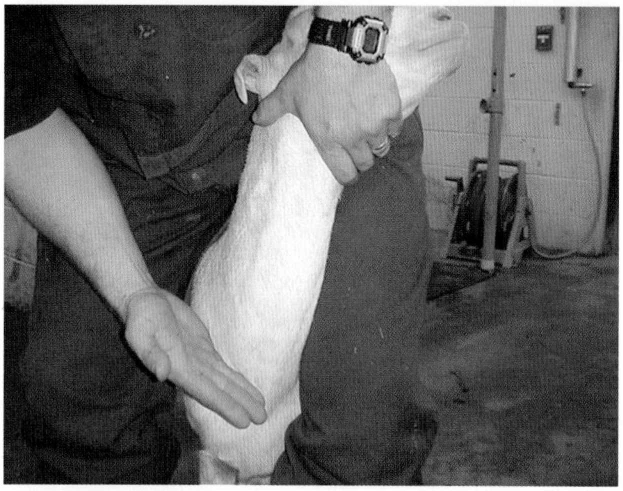

For jugular venipuncture, back the goat into a corner and push it sideways against the wall. Use one hand to hold its head to the side and use the other hand to occlude the vessel.

ORAL MEDICATION

Most medications given to goats are either in a bolus or liquid form. To give the goat a dose of medicine, back it into a corner and, if you are tall enough, straddle it. Hold the drenching syringe in your dominant hand and lift the goat's head with your nondominant hand. Insert the syringe at the commissure of the lips while lifting the goat's head up slightly with your nondominant hand (Fig. 8-8).

FIG. 8-8

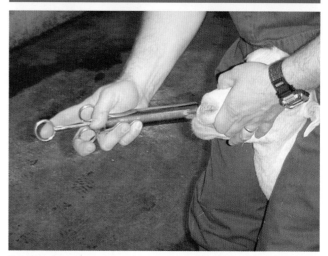

Hold the drenching syringe in your dominant hand and lift the goat's head with your nondominant hand. Insert the syringe at the commissure of the goat's lips while lifting its head up slightly with your nondominant hand.

RESTRAINT FOR HOOF TRIMMING

Restraint for trimming the hooves of a goat is much the same as that used for horses. Have the goat tied or have someone hold the goat using its beard and neck or its cheeks.

To trim the goat's front feet, stand slightly in front of the leg on which you will work. Grasp the leg at the carpus, lift, and gently bend it at the knee. Hold the foot with one hand while trimming with the other because the hooves on a goat are usually soft enough to be trimmed with hoof shears (Fig. 8-9, *A*). Alternatively, you can place the goat's foot on your bent knee or an overturned bucket, freeing both hands. Either technique works well.

Restrain the goat's rear feet by standing beside the rear leg on which you will work. Grasp the leg at the tar-sus, lift, and gently stretch it out behind the goat. Rest the outstretched leg on your bent knee or an overturned bucket so the leg is supported comfortably for the goat (Fig. 8-9, *B*).

RESTRAINT FOR DEHORNING AND CASTRATION

Capture the kid, sit down, and fold its legs down into your lap. Place your forearms on its back to keep it from regaining its feet. Grasp the kid's head by positioning your hands on each side of its neck with your fingers wrapped around its mandible. Place your thumbs behind the kid's ears so that after you have removed the horns you can place your thumbs over the wounds to apply pressure. Restraint for castration is the same as that used for the lamb (see Chapter 7).

FIG. 8-9

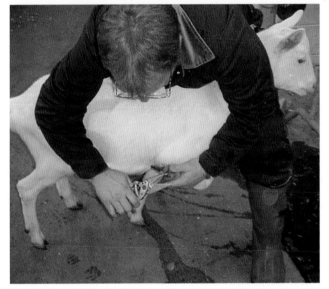

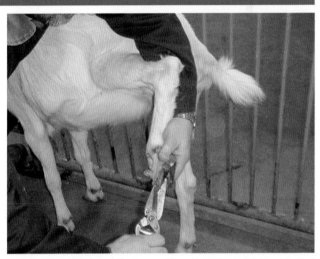

A You can hold the goat's foot with one hand while trimming with the other, because the hooves on a goat are usually soft enough to be trimmed with hoof shears.

B Grasp the goat's leg at the tarsus, lift, and gently stretch it out behind the goat. Rest the outstretched leg on your bent knee or an overturned bucket so the leg is supported comfortably for the goat.

SUGGESTED READINGS

Edwards LM: Behavior and diseases of the dairy goat, *Vet Tech* 4:294–300, 1983.

Fowler ME: *Restraint and handling of wild and domestic animals*, Ames, IA, 1978, Iowa State University Press, 135–138.

Leahy JR, Barrow P: *Restraint of animals*, Ithaca, NY, 1953, Cornell Campus Store, 237–244.

Sonsthagen TF: *Restraint of domestic animals*, St. Louis, 1991, Mosby.

Todd-Jenkins K, Dugan B, Remsburg DW, Montgomery C: Restraint and handling of animals. In *McCurnin's clinical textbook for veterinary technicians*, ed 8, Philadelphia, 2014, Saunders.

9

Restraint of Swine

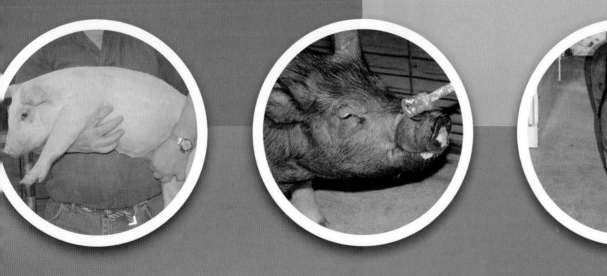

Pigs are generally intelligent, stubborn, contrary, vocal, and sometimes downright vicious animals. These traits make the pig one of the most difficult animals to restrain without injury to you or to the pig. Though pigs seem like hardy animals, they have some physical disadvantages. Poor eyesight makes them easily frightened. An insulating layer of fat makes them susceptible to hyperthermia if treated too roughly for long periods. Their small-boned legs can break easily if grasped or tied in the wrong manner. For this reason, you must move slowly and deliberately when handling pigs. Talk to reassure the animals, and handle them as gently as possible.

A pig's primary means of defense is its sharp teeth, which even in newborn pigs can cause much damage. A pig's snout and shoulder and neck muscles are very strong, allowing it to lift heavy panels of fencing or push you into the fence or ground.

With their streamlined bodies, pigs can squeeze through small openings. This can be quite dangerous if a pig is angry and lifts fence panels and squeezes through openings to chase you. The pig's streamlined body also makes it difficult to hold it with bare hands, so ropes or other restraint tools must be used. Working quickly, quietly, and efficiently minimizes the possibility of injury to you and the pig.

MOVING AND CAPTURING PIGS

It is nearly impossible to capture one pig out of a herd because pigs cannot be herded like cows or sheep. Other pigs may come to the aid of a squealing herd mate, and they may become aggressive without much warning.

HURDLES

The safest method for capturing a single pig from a herd is to move all of the pigs into a small pen using barriers or hurdles. Hurdles are flat, solid pieces of wood, plastic, or metal large enough to cover your legs. Some are equipped with handles or holes cut into them so you can easily carry them in front of you (Fig. 9-1, *A*). Hurdles are solid because if a pig can see through a hurdle it will attempt to go through or under it. You can use a hurdle to turn a pig by simply setting the hurdle in front or to the side of the pig's head (Fig. 9-1, *B*). The pigs will believe they have just run up to a wall and will turn in the opposite direction (Fig. 9-1, *C*). Hurdles can be used to crowd the pigs into a pen or to set up temporary fences while the pigs are moved from place to place. They are also used to

FIG. 9-1

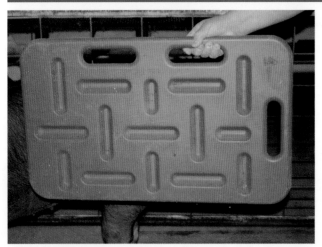

A Hurdles are flat, solid pieces of wood, plastic, or metal large enough to cover your legs.

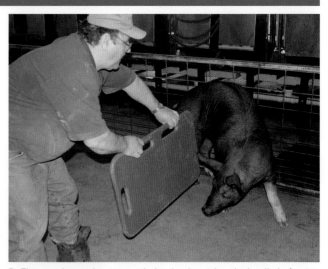

B They can be used to turn a pig by simply setting the hurdle in front or to the side of the pig's head.

(**Figure 9-1,** continued on following page)

FIG. 9-1 cont.

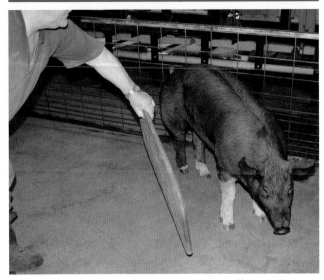

C The pig believes it has just run up to a wall and will turn in the opposite direction.

isolate a particular pig after the herd has been moved into a smaller pen. If a pig tries to go under the hurdle, pull the top of the hurdle toward you.

PADDLES

Pigs can be directed forward with a flat stick or paddle (Fig. 9-2, *A*). Gently tapping the pig on the shoulder, rump, or side of the face turns the animal in the desired direction (Fig. 9-2, *B*). Do not use the paddle to inflict pain because you can enrage the pig and it may come after you. You may also damage its body with severe blows, causing carcass bruising. If you slap the pig on the snout to stop its forward momentum, be careful not to slap it too hard, which can have the opposite effect by angering the animal so it becomes aggressive. Before working with a pig or group of pigs, plan possible escape routes you can use if a pig becomes aggressive.

BUCKET

If a paddle or hurdle is not available, you can place a bucket over the pig's head to move it to a particular place. The pig naturally backs away from the bucket. By holding onto the tail and steering the pig, you move the animal as needed. The trick is to keep the bucket on the pig's head.

FIG. 9-2

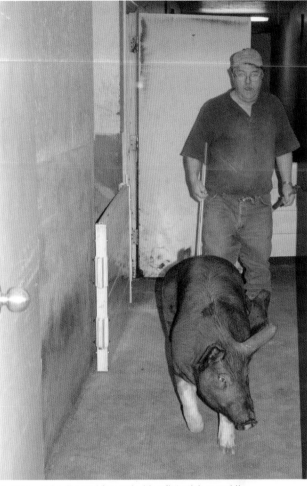

A Pigs can be directed forward with a flat stick or paddle.

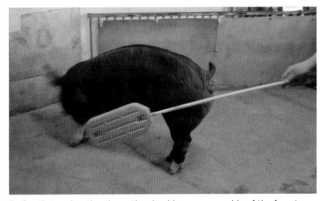

B Gently tapping the pig on the shoulder, rump, or side of the face turns the animal in the desired direction.

CARRYING OR LIFTING PIGS

Pigs weighing less than 50 lbs can be restrained for vaccination, castration, or the administration of medication by lifting them by the rear feet. To restrain for castration or axillary and inguinal vaccination, capture the pig by a rear leg proximal to the hock. Grasp a rear leg in each hand and lift the body, placing the head between your legs (Fig. 9-3, *A*). Let the pig's front legs touch the ground to support some of the animal's weight and to help calm it. If the vaccination is to be given behind the ear or on the shoulder, or if medication is to be given orally, catch the pig in the same manner but elevate its front legs off the ground, letting the animal's shoulders and back rest against your legs for support.

You can quickly lift newborn pigs by the tail. With older piglets up to 4 lbs include a rear leg in your grasp to prevent tail injury. Grasp piglets that weigh more than 4 lbs by a rear leg. Then quickly place one hand under the pig's chest and the other over its flank. Holding piglets firmly but gently in this manner usually calms them and stops their squealing (Fig. 9-3, *B*). This works as well on older pigs.

Be prepared to move quickly if the piglets squeal and the sow is near. A sow with a litter should be assumed to be aggressive. She may try to climb over the farrowing crate or go under it to come to the defense of her squealing piglets. For this reason it is best to move the piglets to another room to work on them.

FIG. 9-3

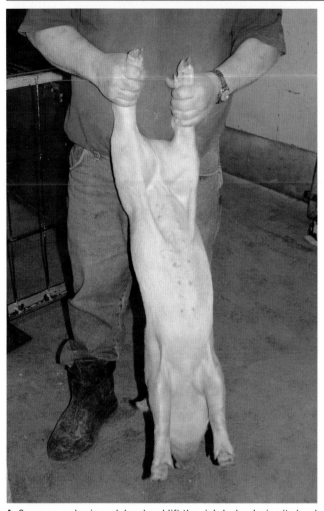

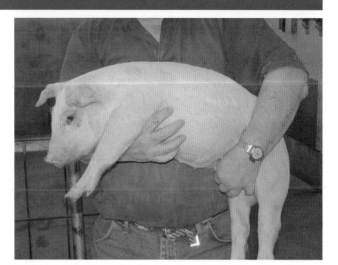

B Then quickly place one hand under the pig's chest and the other over the flank holding the body close.

A Grasp a rear leg in each hand and lift the pig's body, placing its head between your legs.

RESTRAINT OF THE HEAD

Most of the restraint procedures on adult pigs involve the head. Because the pig is such a predictably stubborn creature, you can use its stubbornness to your advantage. Pigs naturally move in a direction opposite to the one in which they are steered. By pulling or pushing in the opposite direction, you can usually make a pig move in the desired direction.

HOG SNARE

A hog snare is the restraint tool of choice when restraining a large pig. The snare is usually a metal pipe with a cable loop on one end. The free end of the cable runs through the hollow pipe so the size of the loop can be controlled. Dangle the loop in front of the pig (Fig. 9-4, *A*). When the pig mouths the loop, push it into the animal's mouth behind its tusks to the commissure of its lips and tighten the loop (Fig. 9-4, *B*). Be ready for an adverse reaction and move with the pig as the cable moves into the mouth (Fig. 9-4, *C*). It may whip its head around trying to dislodge the cable. Be careful not to apply excessive pressure to the pig's snout because the cable may damage it. After you have tightened the cable around the pig's snout, lean away from the pig, keeping your arms up close to your chest (Fig. 9-4, *D*). Keep your arms tucked in so that if the pig does decide to fight you will not be pulled off balance. Usually a pig will lean back as well and stop swinging its head (Fig. 9-4, *E*). After you have finished the procedure, release the pig by pushing down on the handle and quickly moving the snare out of the pig's mouth (Fig. 9-4, *F*). This is especially important if the pig has tusks. If the snare becomes caught on the tusks, it most likely will be jerked out of your hands and the pig may swing its head violently to get rid of it. This makes the snare a dangerous object, not only as it is swung about but also when it does finally come loose and becomes a deadly flying object that is going to leave a mark if it hits you.

Be prepared for loud squealing as you catch and hold the pig (actually it is more of a scream than a squeal). The pig may not fight the snare but it will not be too happy about it and will let everyone in the county know that something has caught it. Ear protection is highly recommended for both the handler and the veterinary personnel when performing this restraint procedure.

The hog snare should be in place only for 20 to 30 minutes; after that the snout loses feeling and the snare will not be as effective. Venipuncture, physical examinations, and injections are just some of the procedures done on a pig that is being held by a snare.

FIG. 9-4

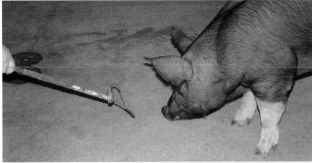

A The loop is dangled in front of the pig.

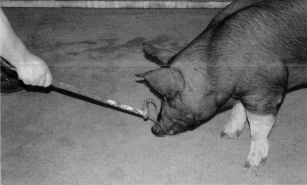

B When the pig mouths the loop, push it into the pig's mouth behind its tusks to the commissure of the lips, and tighten the loop.

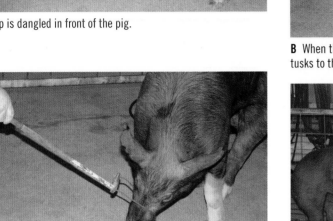

C Be ready for an adverse reaction and move with the pig as the cable moves into the mouth.

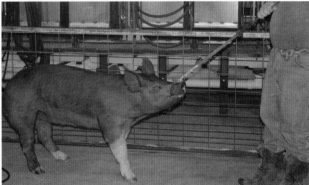

D After the cable is tightened around the pig's snout, lean away from the pig, keeping your arms up close to your chest.

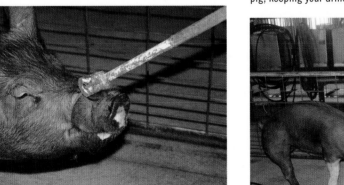

E Usually the pig will lean back as well and stop swinging its head.

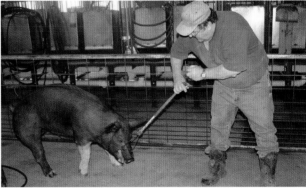

F To release the pig, push down on the handle and quickly move the snare out of its mouth.

SNUBBING ROPE

A snubbing rope works well if you need to tie a pig to a fence. Make a loop in a length of rope by tying a slipknot and making it into a small loop, then running the end through that loop to make a bigger loop that can come undone when the pressure is released. Stand close behind the pig and dangle the loop in front of the animal's face. When the pig begins to mouth the rope, quickly pull the loop into the pig's mouth as close to the commissure of the lips as possible and tighten it across the top of the pig's snout. The rope must be behind the tusks and this may be difficult to accomplish on a boar with large tusks.

If the pig will not mouth the rope, force the loop into the pig's mouth by grasping both sides of the loop and sawing the rope back and forth. Once the rope is in the pig's mouth, apply steady pressure and move to the front of the pig. The animal will naturally pull against this forward pressure, so you will have to loop the rope around the post and take up slack as the pig moves forward. Tie the rope with a halter tie to a vertical post that is set well into the ground or concrete. The pig will back away from the rope and could potentially pull a fence down or break horizontal boards. Do not leave the rope on for more than 15 to 20 minutes because of its tourniquet-like effect on the snout. Do not leave the animal unattended because it may chew through the rope. If a pig violently resists a single rope, you can place another snubbing rope into the pig's mouth and the pig can be cross-tied.

WHOLE-BODY RESTRAINT

TROUGH

A restraint tool that can be used to keep smaller pigs on their backs is a V-shaped trough (Fig. 9-5, *A*). Place the pig in the trough on its back (Fig. 9-5, *B*). Hold its front feet down and stretch its neck out for a venipuncture. If you are going to perform surgery on the pig, tie a small-diameter rope around the pig's feet, run the rope to the sides of the trough, and tie it in a quick-release knot. This keeps the pig in place so that you can tilt the trough in any direction.

HOBBLES

There are various ways to cast pigs. All involve initially gaining control of the pig's head with a snubbing rope or snare. After securing the snubbing rope to the pig's snout, use a half hitch to secure one of the pig's rear legs. Now pull the rope to draw the pig's foot and nose together, knocking the animal off its feet.

Another method is to attach a rope to a front and rear leg on one side of the pig. Pass both ropes under the pig's abdomen and up the opposite side of the pig and then over the back, toward you. Pulling up on the ropes pulls the pig's feet out from under it, toppling it over on its side. Use the ropes to tie its legs together.

FIG. 9-5

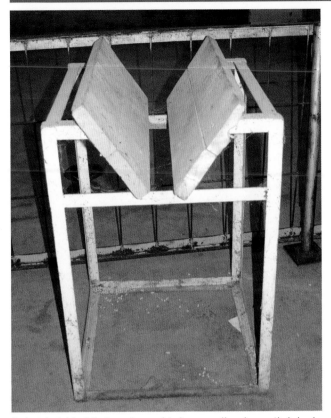

A A restraint tool that can be used to keep smaller pigs on their backs is a V-shaped trough.

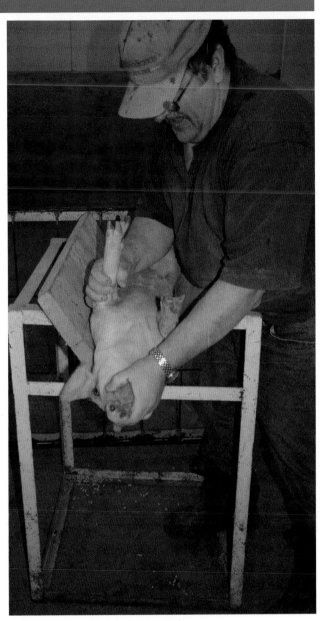

B Place the pig in the trough on its back.

SUGGESTED READINGS

Fowler ME: *Restraint and handling of wild and domestic animals*, Ames, IA, 1978, Iowa State University Press.

Kocab JM: Restraint of pigs, *New Methods*: 12–13, February 1983.

Leahy JR, Barrow P: *Restraint of animals*, Ithaca, NY, 1953, Cornell Campus Store.

Sonsthagen TF: *Restraint of domestic animals*, St. Louis, 1991, Mosby.

Todd-Jenkins K, Dugan B, Remsburg DW, Montgomery C: Restraint and handling of animals. In *McCurnin's clinical textbook for veterinary technicians*, ed 8, Philadelphia, 2014, Saunders.

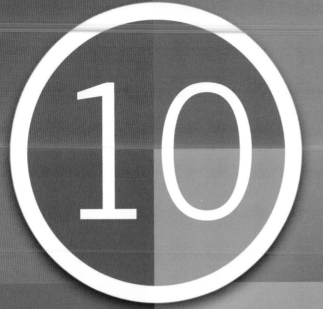

Restraint of Rodents, Rabbits, and Ferrets

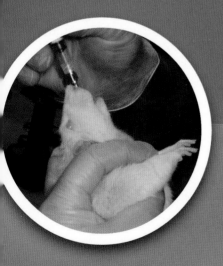
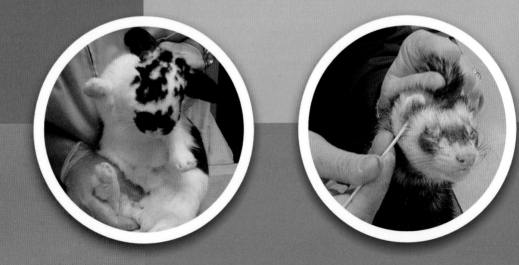

Working with rodents, rabbits, and ferrets can be a fun and rewarding experience. Not only are these species used commonly in research animal medicine, they are increasingly being seen in veterinary clinics for medical and surgical treatments. As people's lives have become busier and constraints on their time greater, many have turned to these smaller species as beloved family pets, often affording them high-quality veterinary care. The job of providing quality nursing care then falls upon the veterinary professional. To ensure good care, proper handling and restraint is of utmost importance so that you do not harm the animal by the intended treatment. Take care to handle these small animals gently to reduce their stress. Though we tend to think of these animals as a group, it is important to remember they are individuals and have unique behaviors and special needs. By knowing the anatomy, special needs, and behaviors of each species, we can reduce the risks when handling them. Be sure to pay attention to the details when you have completed the procedures.

There are several ways to improve the encounter and ensure success when working with these species: (1) learn the behaviors of the species to better anticipate how the animal may react to a procedure, (2) explore appropriate ways to handle and restrain these species for a given procedure, (3) have all needed equipment and supplies ready before starting procedures to minimize restraint times, and (4) carefully examine and employ the handling and restraint techniques used by someone who has experience working with these species. In addition, it is a good practice to wear examination gloves when working with the rodent species. Exposure to rodents may lead to allergies, so prevention starts with your personal protection.

Note that the veterinary professional should use aseptic techniques while completing injections for any of these animals. You can readily accomplish this by swabbing an injection site with a cleansing agent (e.g., 70% isopropyl alcohol) to prepare the injection site as well as using a sterile needle and syringe. Although some may consider these animals as having less value, they are still beloved pets or valuable research animals, so always take care to prevent disease.

THE MOUSE

More and more families are keeping mice as pets. Mice are small and easy to care for, require little space, and generally do not cost a lot. Routine veterinary care for mice includes nail trims, teeth checks and trims, and routine physical examinations. In addition, a veterinary professional may be asked to administer medications and collect blood samples.

Mice are shy creatures that like to be with other mice in dark areas of their cage. Mice avoid bright lights and loud sounds and, generally, the less you handle them, the calmer they will remain. It is worth the time spent to plan ahead before starting any procedures, so get all your supplies ready before handling and restraint. Because of the small size of mice, you must be careful not to hold them too tightly or you may crush them. To prevent the mouse from becoming stressed from mishandling and biting you, control it by grasping its scruff and hold the base of its tail in one hand.

CAGE RETRIEVAL AND RESTRAINT

After removing the top of the cage, reach in and quickly grasp the mouse firmly at the most proximal portion (base) of the tail (Fig. 10-1, *A*). Never grab the tail in the distal two thirds of the tail; it is possible to deglove the tissue from the mouse's vertebrae. Lift the mouse carefully by the base of its tail to the top of the cage or a flat surface so that it can gain footing (Fig. 10-1, *B*). Once the mouse has secured its footing and while you are still holding its tail, push down and slide your fingers from caudal to cranial along the spine to get access to its scruff. Firmly grasp its scruff just caudal to its ears between your thumb and index finger. Be sure to gather enough skin between your fingers and be sure you are not too far caudal (Fig. 10-1, *C*). This prevents the mouse from being able to move its head so that it can injure itself or bite you. Then lift the mouse so that its body is in the palm of your hand and your little finger is wrapped around its tail. Using this restraint, you can trim nails, check and trim teeth, and perform necessary medical procedures (Fig. 10-1, *D*).

FIG. 10-1

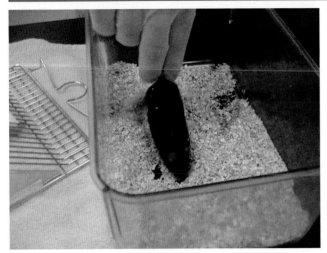

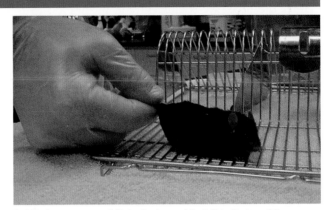

B Lift the mouse carefully by the base of its tail to the top of the cage or a flat surface so that it can gain its footing.

A After removing the top of the cage, reach in and quickly grasp the mouse firmly at the most proximal portion (base) of its tail.

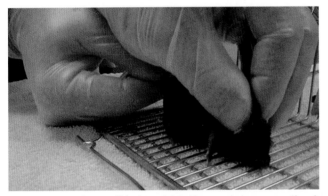

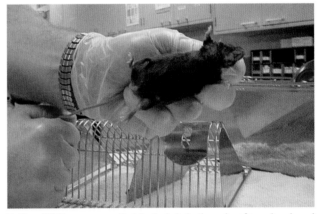

D Then lift the mouse so that its body is in the palm of your hand, and wrap your little finger around its tail to hold its body firmly in the palm of your hand.

C Firmly grasp the scruff just caudal to the ears between your thumb and index finger.

ORAL GAVAGE

Gather the necessary equipment and medication to be administered via gavage. The gavage needle for the mouse is a 20-gauge by 2-inch stainless steel needle with a round ball tip (Fig. 10-2, *A*). When prepared, pick the mouse up as described in Fig. 10-1, *A* to *D*. Hold the mouse in your nondominant hand. Be sure that you can fully extend its head and neck (Fig. 10-2, *B*). Begin by placing the gavage needle gently into the mouse's diastema (the space just caudal to its incisors where it has no teeth). Once you have placed the needle into the animal's mouth you must fully extend its head and neck so that you can insert the gavage needle down the esophagus and not the trachea

(Fig. 10-2, *C*). As you insert the needle, you may notice slight resistance to its forward placement when entering the mouse's esophagus. Do not force the needle too hard at this point, or you may rupture the delicate mucosal lining in the oropharynx. As long as the mouse's head is fully extended, you will find placement of the gavage needle rather easy. Once the full length of the needle is in place, you will note that the needle hub will be just in the mouse's mouth (Fig. 10-2, *D*). At this point, the medication can be administered. If the needle is in the mouse's trachea, the needle will not go in as far. Aspiration before delivery is not necessary because correct needle placement indicates correct location.

FIG. 10-2

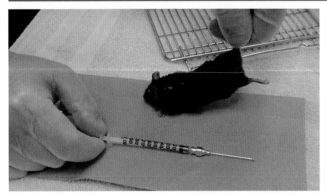

A The gavage needle for the mouse is a 20-gauge by 2-inch stainless steel needle with a round ball tip.

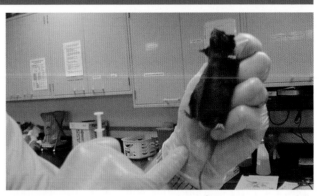

B Hold the mouse in your nondominant hand. Be sure that you can fully extend its head and neck.

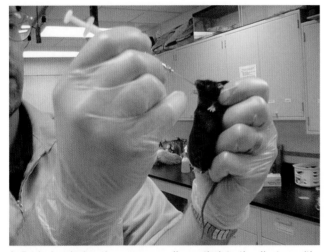

C Begin by placing the gavage needle gently into the diastema (the space just caudal to its incisors where it has no teeth).

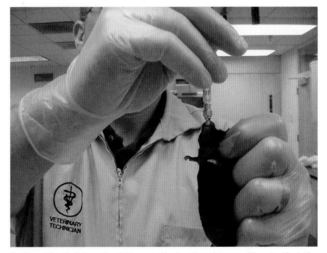

D Once the full length of the needle is placed, you will note that the needle hub will be just in the animal's mouth.

INJECTIONS

You can give subcutaneous injections by holding the mouse by its scruff just caudal to its ears while allowing it to stand on a firm tabletop with good footing. Bring the needle and syringe in a cranial to caudal direction to the mouse's head, and place the needle into the tent you have created in the scruff. With proper placement, the needle and syringe assist in keeping the mouse's head down while you complete the injection (Fig. 10-3, *A*).

Because of the small size of the caudal thigh muscles in the mouse, intramuscular injection is not recommended. However, if you must use this route to deliver medications, use extra caution while completing the injection. While holding the mouse as described in Fig. 10-1, *D*, the restrainer can use a two-hand approach, holding the animal's tail in his or her second hand. The person who will administer the injection then identifies the location of the femur by palpation and places the needle into the muscles of the mouse's thigh so that the needle angles away from its femur (Fig. 10-3, *B*). This will decrease the chance of irritation to the mouse's ischiatic nerve.

The intraperitoneal injection in the mouse is ideal for delivery of numerous injectables, including antibiotics, anesthetics, and euthanasia solutions. Hold the mouse as described in Fig. 10-1, *D*. Then tip the mouse so that its head is lower than its abdomen (Fig. 10-3, *C*). This will cause the gastrointestinal tract to fall toward the diaphragm and away from your injection site. Then locate the animal's stifles and choose an injection site in the lower left (or right) quadrant of its abdomen (Fig. 10-3, *D*). Place the needle quickly through the skin and musculature of the abdomen at a 30-degree angle (Fig. 10-3, *E*). Aspirate to ensure you do not see gastrointestinal contents (brown), urine (clear yellow), or blood. Seeing any of these indicates incorrect placement, and you should start the injection again in a different location. If nothing is aspirated, you may complete the injection.

FIG. 10-3

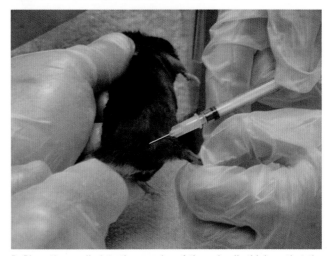

A With proper placement, the needle and syringe assist in keeping the mouse's head down while you complete the injection.

B Place the needle into the muscles of the animal's thigh so that the needle angles away from its femur.

(**Figure 10-3,** continued on following page)

FIG. 10-3 cont.

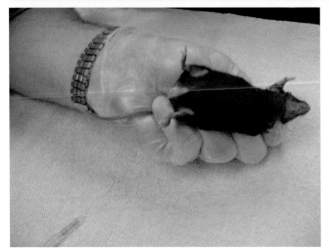

C Tip the mouse so that its head is lower than its abdomen.

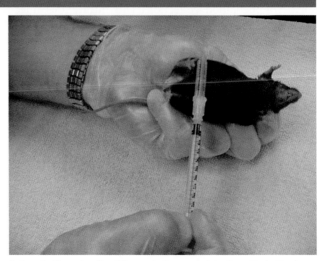

D Locate the animal's stifles and choose an injection site in the lower left (or right) quadrant of its abdomen.

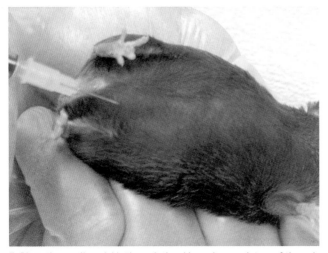

E Place the needle quickly through the skin and musculature of the animal's abdomen at a 30-degree angle.

The lateral tail veins of the mouse can be used for small-volume blood collections and intravenous injections. Because of the small size of the vein, it takes a fair bit of skill and patience to use the vein consistently. However, as with other procedures, there are steps you can take to improve your success. First of all, adequate restraint is the key. Mice can be held by an assistant, placed in a commercial plastic rodent restrainer or polyvinylchloride (PVC) tubing, or even placed in a plastic bag restrainer as long as you have access to the tail vein to complete the venipuncture. Beyond restraint, it is also important to adequately warm the tail to dilate the tail veins. Placing the whole mouse or just the mouse's tail in close proximity to a heating lamp or other warming device for 5 minutes will often suffice. Then properly restrain the animal in a way that allows access to the lateral tail veins (Fig. 10-4). Proximal occlusion of the vessel is necessary and can be completed by hand, or you can use a rubber band and hemostat, which can be applied as a tourniquet. Once you can visualize the tail vein, approach at a shallow angle parallel to the vessel and thread the needle carefully. Aspirate to ensure placement, then complete the venipuncture as done with other animals. Remember that success comes with practice.

FIG. 10-4

Properly restrain the animal in a way that allows access to the lateral tail veins.

THE RAT

Many people are finding that rats make good companions that can be housed easily in apartments or small houses. They require little daily care, and they can learn to enjoy human companionship enormously. They are intelligent animals that make excellent pets and can be trained quickly. They are curious and gentle but easily startled. When handling a rat, move slowly and give it time to adjust to you. When threatened or frightened, a rat's natural instinct is to run and hide, not to bite you. If cornered, however, a rat will bite as a last resort. While handling rats, wear examination gloves to prevent you from developing allergies. Smock pockets are often quiet places the rat loves, and placing it in your smock pocket in between procedures will often calm it down. Routine veterinary procedures that should be included in a rat's health maintenance program include nail trims, teeth checks and trims as needed, and general physical examinations. A veterinary professional may also be asked to help restrain a rat for administration of medication or blood collection.

Approach the rat to remove it from its cage in a calm, confident manner. Do not corner the rat and threaten it by approaching directly at its head. Instead, approach the rat with your hand over its back, coming from its tail. Grab the base of the rat's tail firmly, pick the rat up, and transport it to the cage top or table (Fig. 10-5, A). While holding the base of its tail, bring your hand over the animal's shoulders so that you can slide your fingers around its mandible and restrain its head. Your fingers should support its mandible on both sides, but be sure not to wrap your fingers around the animal's trachea. One method of restraint is to use your thumb to support one side of the animal's mandible and your index finger to support the other while your middle finger wraps around the animal's axilla (armpit) (Fig. 10-5, B).

FIG. 10-5

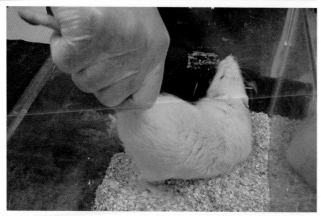

A Grab the base of the rat's tail firmly and pick up the rat and transport it to the cage top or table.

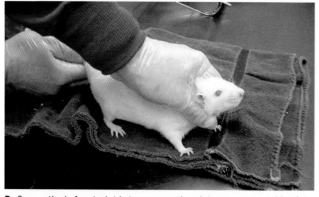

B One method of restraint is to use your thumb to support one side of the animal's mandible and your index finger to support the other while your middle finger wraps around the animal's axilla.

FIG. 10-6

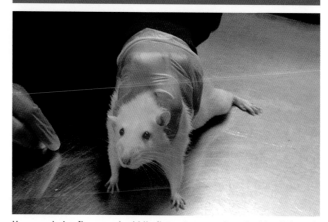

Use your index finger and middle finger to support each side of the animal's mandible while your thumb and ring finger surround the animal's axilla (armpits).

Another method of restraint is to use your index finger and middle finger to support each side of the animal's mandible while your thumb and ring finger surround the animal's axilla (Fig. 10-6). Which method you use will depend on the size of your hand and the size of the rat.

FIG. 10-7

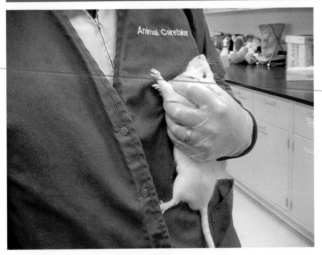

A Hold the rat firmly against your body.

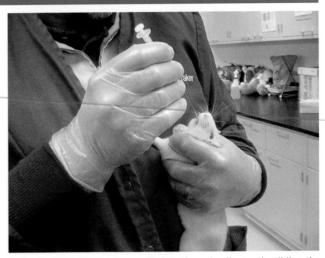

B Gently place the gavage needle into the animal's mouth, sliding the tip of the needle into its mouth at the diastema (the space just caudal to the incisors where there are no teeth).

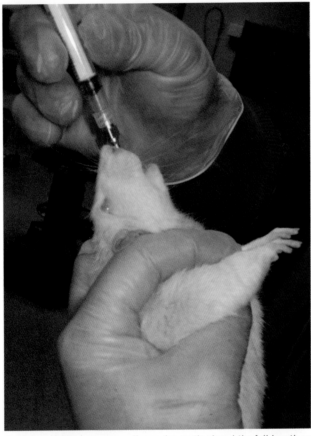

C As long as the gavage needle can be gently placed the full length so that the hub is to the animal's mouth, placement is correct.

ORAL GAVAGE

To administer oral medication to a rat, it is best to gavage the animal. The gavage needle for the rat is an 18-gauge by 3-inch stainless steel needle with a round ball tip. The proper restraint and extension of the animal's head and neck are of utmost importance to ensure proper placement of the gavage needle and prevent esophageal perforation or improper placement in the trachea. To start, hold the rat firmly against your body (Fig. 10-7, *A*) Place your fingers around the mandible so that you will be able to extend the rat's head and neck. Gently place the gavage needle into the animal's mouth, sliding the tip of the needle into the mouth at the diastema (the space just caudal to the incisors where there are no teeth) (Fig. 10-7, *B*). Be sure to extend the animal's head and neck as you gently advance the gavage needle. While advancing the gavage needle down the esophagus, there should be slight resistance. If the needle advances with no resistance or you cannot place the needle the full length to the hub, you are likely to be in the trachea. As long as the gavage needle can be placed the full length so the hub is to the animal's mouth, placement is correct (Fig. 10-7, *C*). At this point you can administer the medication. As with the mouse, aspiration before delivery is not necessary because correct needle placement indicates correct location.

INJECTIONS

In the rat, you can administer parenteral medications by subcutaneous, intramuscular, or intraperitoneal routes. To administer a subcutaneous injection, place the rat on a firm tabletop. Provide a towel or surface that allows the rat to gain footing. Firmly hold the rat over the scapular area while creating a subcutaneous tent. Bring the needle and syringe directly over the animal's head in a cranial to caudal direction so that it rests gently on its head and the needle can enter the subcutaneous tent you have created (Fig. 10-8).

To administer an intramuscular injection to a rat, two people are involved, with the restrainer holding the rat in a laterally recumbent position. Use the restraint discussed in Figs. 10-5, *B*, and 10-6; in addition, hold the base of the animal's tail while supporting the rat against the arm of the person restraining the rat. The person administering the injection will then carefully locate the animal's femur by palpating. Once the femur has been located, the injection can be administered so that the needle is placed parallel and caudal to the femur to avoid hitting the ischiatic nerve (Fig. 10-9).

FIG. 10-8

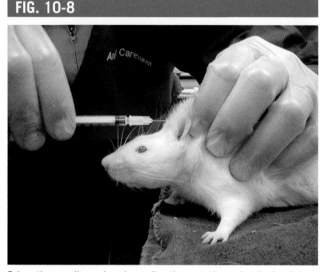

Bring the needle and syringe directly over the animal's head in a cranial-to-caudal direction so that it rests gently on the animal's head and the needle can enter the subcutaneous tent that you have created.

FIG. 10-9

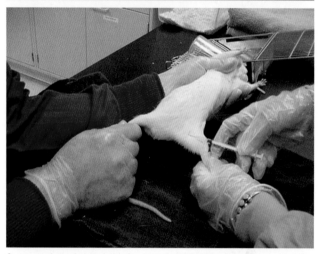

Once you have located the femur, administer the injection so that the needle is parallel and caudal to the femur to avoid hitting the animal's ischiatic nerve.

The intraperitoneal injection is used to deliver fluids as well as certain medications to rats. The rat should be held against your body so that its head is lower than its abdomen. This allows its gastrointestinal tract to fall toward the head and away from your injection site. With the heel of your hand, pin the rat's head against your body and rotate its body away from you to expose its abdomen (Fig. 10-10, *A*). The syringe in Fig. 10-10, *B*, demonstrates the level at which you will give the injection. Needle placement should be in the lower right quadrant of the animal's abdomen with the needle pointing cranially. The needle should be placed with a quick motion so that it pops through the skin and abdominal muscles. Avoid puncturing the abdomen too slowly, as you are more likely to trap the animal's intestine this way (Fig. 10-10, *C*). Intraperitoneal injections can also be performed using the same anatomic landmarks as described but utilizing a two-person method (Fig. 10-10, *D*).

FIG. 10-10

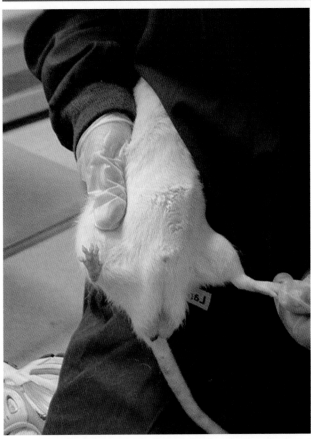

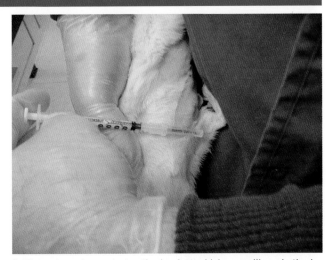

B The syringe demonstrates the level at which you will apply the injection. Needle placement should be in the lower right quadrant of the animal's abdomen with the needle pointing cranially.

A With the heel of your hand, pin the rat's head against your body and rotate its body away from you to expose its abdomen.

(**Figure 10-10,** continued on following page)

FIG. 10-10 cont.

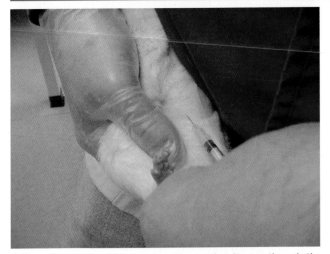

C Place the needle with a quick motion so that it pops through the animal's skin and abdominal muscles.

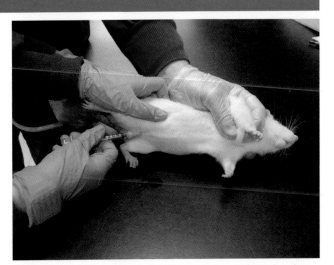

D Alternative intraperitoneal injection can be performed using a two-person method.

BLOOD COLLECTION

Small-volume blood collection can be completed in a rat by using the lateral tail veins. The rat can be restrained in a plastic rat restrainer, which allows easy access to the tail. A plastic bag can also be used for restraint. Simply cut a small hole in one corner, allow the rat to poke its nose out of the hole, then roll the bag up around it so that its tail is protruding. A rubber band and hemostat then function as a tourniquet (Fig. 10-11, *A*). The tail veins are located on either lateral aspect of the animal's tail. Good visualization of these veins is important, so it is often necessary to warm the tail to dilate the veins. Once you can readily locate the animal's lateral tail vein, brace the tail along your hand for support while placing the needle and slowly aspirate blood into the syringe (Fig. 10-11, *B*).

FIG. 10-11

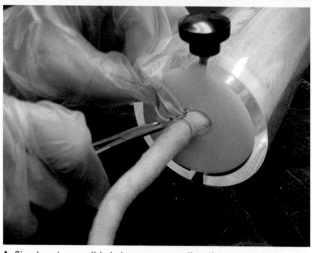 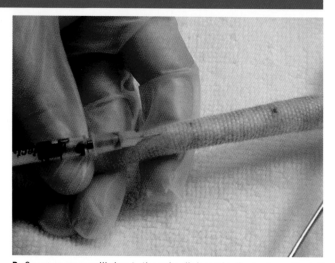

A Simply cut a small hole in one corner, allow the rat to poke his nose out of the hole, then roll the bag up around the animal so that its tail is protruding. A rubber band and hemostat then function as a tourniquet.

B Once you can readily locate the animal's lateral tail vein, brace the tail along your hand for support while placing the needle, and slowly aspirate blood into the syringe.

THE HAMSTER

Hamsters are nocturnal desert animals that are slow to awaken during daylight hours. When attempting to retrieve the hamster, take care not to startle it. Take a few moments to gently and carefully prod the animal until it is awake. Hamsters are known for their "bite now, ask questions later" behavior when being handled. Be sure to gather all needed equipment before removing the hamster from its primary enclosure and handle it as quietly as possible. If you are doing more than simply moving a hamster from cage to cage, you will need to maintain a firm grip on its scruff to prevent it from biting. Generally, hamsters should be housed alone or in well-established pairs to prevent fighting. In addition, hamsters are known to chew on caging unless provided with suitable alternatives.

Hamsters are easily startled, so approach the animal slowly before handling it. Touch a sleeping hamster on its back to allow it to wake up before handling (Fig. 10-12, *A*). One method for retrieving a friendly hamster is to cup the animal in the palm of both hands and transport it to a table surface (Fig. 10-12, *B*). An alternative method to "cupping" the hamster can be used if you are unsure whether the hamster is friendly or if it makes threatening motions toward you. Simply grasp the hamster's scruff behind the head close to its ears and transport it to a table surface covered with a towel (Fig. 10-12, *C*). Take note of the large amounts of loose skin on the hamster.

Once you have moved the hamster out of the cage to a table surface, control the animal by gathering as much of the loose skin as possible at its head and along its back and carefully but firmly pressing the animal to the towel (Fig. 10-12, *D*). Continue to gather all loose skin from cranial to caudal in the palm of your hand, ending with a fistful of loose skin firmly pulled into the palm of your hand (Fig. 10-12, *E*). Be sure you gather adequate skin near the animal's head; otherwise the hamster may be able to turn and bite you. Note the finished restraint hold in Fig. 10-12, *F* and *G*, with the hamster held in a vertical position.

FIG. 10-12

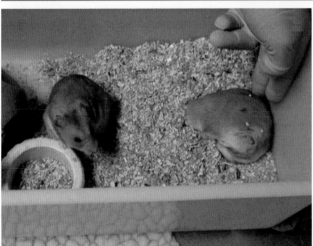

A It is best to touch a sleeping hamster on its back to allow it to wake up before handling.

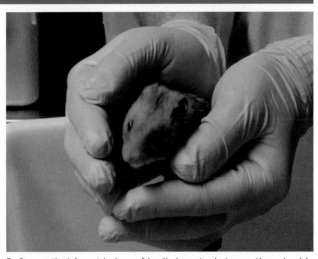

B One method for retrieving a friendly hamster is to cup the animal in the palm of both hands and transport it to a table surface.

(**Figure 10-12**, continued on following page)

FIG. 10-12 cont.

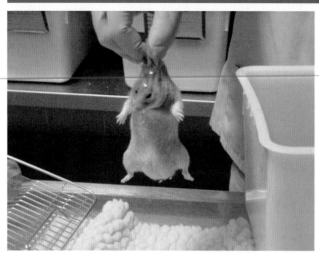

C Simply grasp the hamster's scruff behind its head close to its ears and transport it to a table surface covered with a towel.

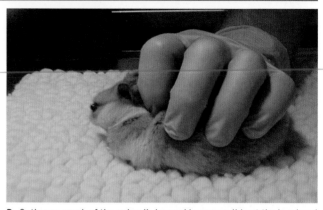

D Gather as much of the animal's loose skin as possible at the head and along the back, and carefully but firmly press the animal to the towel.

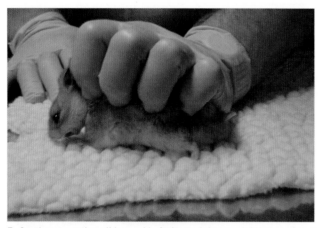

E Continue to gather all loose skin from cranial to caudal in the palm of your hand ending with a fistful of loose skin firmly pulled into the palm of your hand.

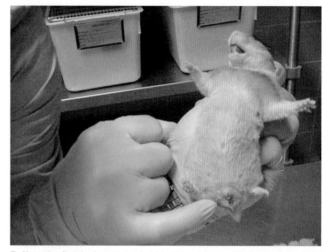

F Note the finished restraint hold in this picture with the hamster held in a vertical position. This is a female hamster.

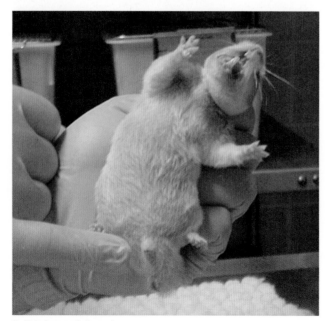

G This is a male hamster.

INJECTIONS

Complete injections in the hamster in much the same manner as used for the mouse. Subcutaneous injections in hamsters should be completed by using the scruff of skin at the base of the animal's neck. While holding the scruff of the hamster, with the animal facing away from you, form a tent of skin (Fig. 10-13, *A*). After cleansing the injection site, bring the needle and syringe in from the caudal aspect of the skin tent, place the needle quickly, and complete the injection (Fig. 10-13, *B*). Complete intramuscular and intraperitoneal injections in the same manner used for the mouse.

FIG. 10-13

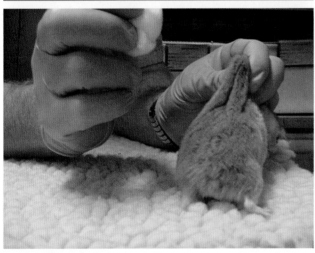

A While holding the hamster's scruff, with the animal facing away from you, form a tent of skin.

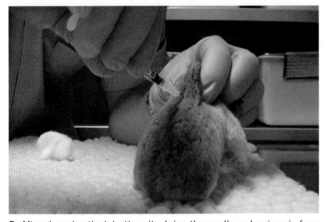

B After cleansing the injection site, bring the needle and syringe in from the caudal aspect of the skin tent, place the needle quickly, and complete the injection.

ORAL GAVAGE

Oral gavage in the hamster can be completed much the same as in the mouse, but with a couple of considerations. Hamsters have large, well-developed cheek pouches that extend from each side of the head and neck to each shoulder. When completing oral gavage in the hamster, place the gavage needle as close to midline as possible to ensure placement down the esophagus and not into one of the animal's extensive cheek pouches.

THE GERBIL

Like the hamster, gerbils are nocturnal desert animals. They are clean, easy-to-handle, easy-to-keep rodents. Gerbils naturally burrow and therefore should be kept in solid caging with bedding that allows them to burrow. They can be easily stressed and become overexcited, which can lead to seizures. You should not lift a gerbil by the tip of its tail, as this may lead to "slipping" of the skin off the tail. It is important when working with gerbils that you have all your supplies ready and keep handling time to a minimum.

Gerbils are curious, social little animals. Before removing a gerbil from its primary enclosure, take a minute to assess its posture, attitude, and stance. Gerbils should take an active interest in you as you approach (Fig. 10-14, *A*). When retrieving the gerbil, reach into its enclosure and

FIG. 10-14

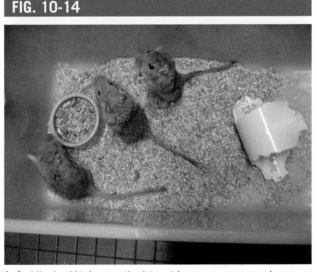

A Gerbils should take an active interest in you as you approach.

(**Figure 10-14,** continued on following page)

bring your hand from over its head to grasp its tail firmly at the base (Fig. 10-14, *B*). Gently lift the animal onto a firm surface, such as the tabletop or cage top. Firmly hold the base of the animal's tail while you scruff the animal with your other hand (Fig. 10-14, *C*). You can then pick the animal up (Fig. 10-14, *D*). Once you have a good hold of the animal's scruff, you can transfer the base of its tail to your little finger on the hand you are scruffing with so that the animal rests in the palm of your hand (Fig. 10-14, *E*).

FIG. 10-14 cont.

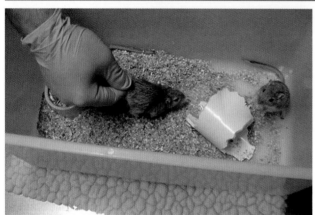

B When retrieving the gerbil, reach into its enclosure, bringing your hand from over its head to grasp its tail firmly at the base.

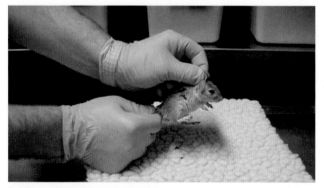

D You can then pick up the animal.

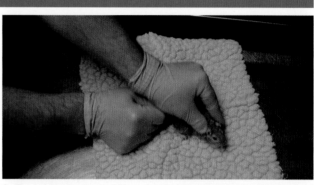

C Firmly hold the base of the animal's tail while you scruff the animal with your other hand.

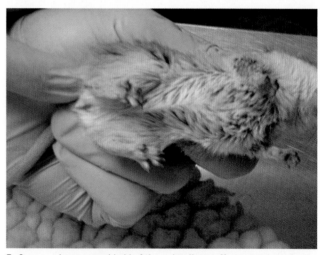

E Once you have a good hold of the animal's scruff, you can transfer the base of its tail to your little finger on the hand you are scruffing with so that the animal rests in the palm of your hand.

INJECTIONS

To administer a subcutaneous injection, swab the tent made in the scruff with alcohol (Fig. 10-15, *A*). Bring the syringe in from a cranial direction while keeping the animal slightly suspended so that its front feet do not have traction while you complete the injection (Fig. 10-15, *B*). As in the mouse and hamster, intramuscular injection is not recommended because of the gerbil's small muscle size; however, you can complete this injection as long as you take extra caution to ensure that you place the needle so as to avoid the ischiatic nerve.

Intraperitoneal injections can be used to deliver fluids to a dehydrated animal. Holding the animal in one hand as previously described, tip the animal's head lower than its body in a dorsally recumbent position. Locate its caudal abdomen and use an alcohol swab to cleanse the area of injection (Fig. 10-16, *A*). The injection should be given to the right (or left) caudal part of the abdomen (Fig. 10-16, *B*). Quickly insert the needle, then aspirate to ensure proper placement and deliver the fluids (Fig. 10-16, *C*).

ORAL GAVAGE

Complete the oral gavage in the gerbil in the same manner used in the mouse. One consideration, however, is that a 20-gauge 2½-inch gavage needle may be necessary to ensure proper placement because of the larger size of the gerbil compared with the mouse.

FIG. 10-15

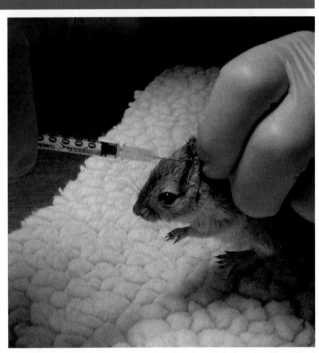

A To administer a subcutaneous injection, swab the tent made in the scruff with alcohol.

B Bring the syringe in from a cranial direction while keeping the animal slightly suspended so that its front feet do not have traction while you are completing the injection.

FIG. 10-16

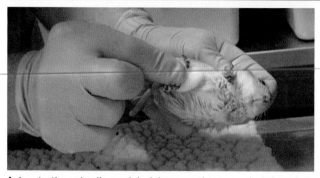

A Locate the animal's caudal abdomen and use an alcohol swab to cleanse the area of injection.

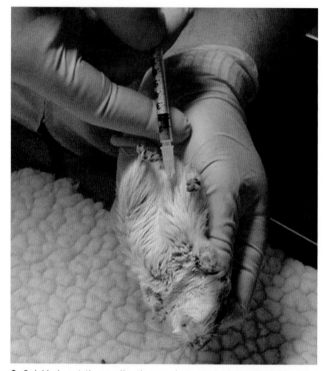

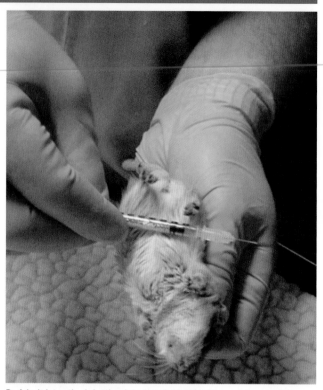

B Administer the injection into the right (or left) caudal part of the animal's abdomen.

C Quickly insert the needle, then aspirate to ensure proper placement and deliver the fluids.

THE GUINEA PIG

Guinea pigs are common pets as well as common research animals. They tend to be social, docile, and quite vocal. Do not be surprised by their vocalizations. They are also shy and timid when removed from their primary housing, and they tend to be active and messy while at home. When startled, guinea pigs will run frantically around their enclosures, so try to work calmly and slowly around them. Routine veterinary care involves nail trims as well as teeth checks and trims. A veterinary professional will also need to know how to administer medication.

To remove a guinea pig from its cage, slowly corner it and place one hand over its head to shield its eyes, and use your other hand to cover the back end (Fig. 10-17, *A*). Guinea pigs are easily scared and become frantic if chased around their cages. Once cornered with their eyes covered, they generally offer little resistance. Always use both hands to remove the guinea pig from its enclosure. Your first hand will continue to cover the animal's eyes and support its head and neck while your other hand scoops and supports its hind end (Fig. 10-17, *B*). You can then lift the guinea pig while supporting its body with your hand (Fig. 10-17, *C*). Since guinea pigs are such shy animals, if your method of restraint allows them to feel that they are hidden, you will have a much easier and safer time. Often it is enough to simply allow the guinea pig to hide in the fold of your arm (Fig. 10-17, *D*).

FIG. 10-17

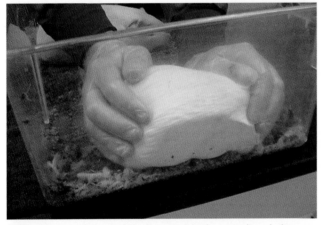

A To remove a guinea pig from its cage, slowly corner it and place one hand over its head to shield its eyes and the other hand to cover the back end.

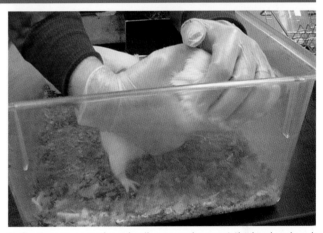

B Continue to cover the animal's eyes and support the head and neck with your first hand, while your other hand scoops and supports the animal's hind end.

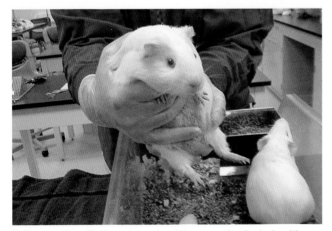

C You can then lift the guinea pig while supporting its body with your hand.

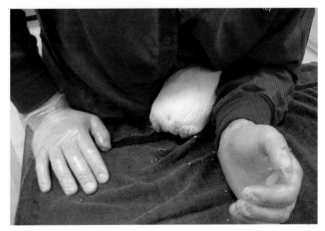

D Restrain it in a way so that it feels it is hidden; you will have an easier and safer time. Often it is enough to simply allow the guinea pig to hide in the fold of your arm.

INJECTIONS

Place the guinea pig on a firm surface with good footing. Cover its eyes with one hand while making a subcutaneous tent of skin just dorsal to its scapulas (Fig. 10-18, *A*). Bring the needle and syringe in caudal to the tent you have made, and quickly insert the needle through the animal's skin (Fig. 10-18, *B*). You will note that the thickness of a guinea pig's skin makes it difficult to penetrate with the needle, so you might need to apply extra force to drive the needle through the skin. As always, aspirate before injection to ensure that you have properly placed the needle before administering the medication.

Intradermal injections are often administered to guinea pigs in research facilities. An area of skin should be shaved on the dorsal aspect of the guinea pig to ensure proper injection technique (Fig. 10-19, *A*). Place the needle into the skin at a 10- to 15-degree angle (Fig. 10-19, *B*). Administration of the medication should provide resistance, and a bleb should form as the medication is administered. Be sure the site you have chosen is readily visible so that you can make observations without further handling the animal.

FIG. 10-18

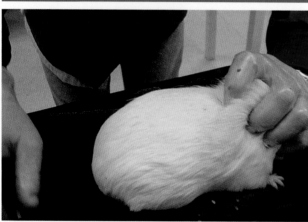

A Place the guinea pig on a firm surface with good footing, and cover its eyes with one hand while making a subcutaneous tent of skin just dorsal to its scapulas.

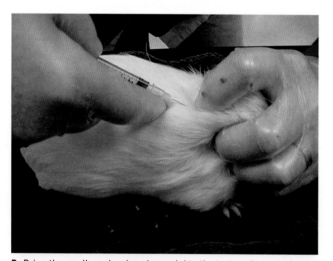

B Bring the needle and syringe in caudal to the tent you have made, and quickly insert the needle through the animal's skin.

FIG. 10-19

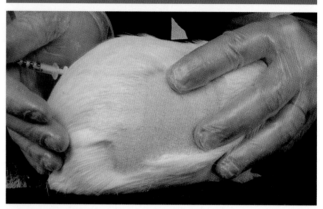

A An area of skin should be shaved on the dorsal aspect of the guinea pig to ensure proper injection technique.

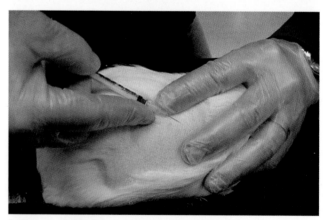

B Place the needle into the skin at a 10- to 15-degree angle.

When completing the intramuscular injection, allow the guinea pig to hide in the crook of your arm so that it feels more comfortable. Be sure you have provided a firm surface for the guinea pig to stand on. The person administering the injection should locate the animal's femur by palpation (Fig. 10-20, *A*). After swabbing the injection site with alcohol, place the needle away from the femur to avoid hitting the animal's ischiatic nerve (Fig. 10-20, *B*).

FIG. 10-20

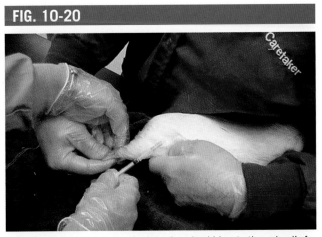

A The person administering the injection should locate the animal's femur by palpation.

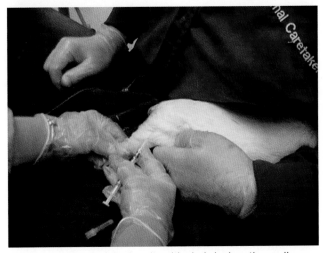

B After swabbing the injection site with alcohol, place the needle away from the animal's femur to avoid hitting its ischiatic nerve.

THE RABBIT

Rabbits are quiet, shy, nocturnal animals and are not generally aggressive to people. Rabbits can easily be frightened, so take care to handle them in a quiet, calm manner. Because of the mass of a rabbit's massive hind limb muscles compared with the relatively small bone mass in the hind limbs, take care to always support a rabbit's hind limbs. If a rabbit gives a quick, powerful kick, it can cause serious damage to its spinal cord, possibly leading to hind limb paralysis. A rabbit can also use its massive hind limbs as a means of escape and protection and can cause severe injury (e.g., deep scratches) to the handler if its back end is not immobilized.

If you can provide a way for the rabbit to feel it is hiding, you can often provide a calmer, safer working situation. One method is to shield the rabbit's eyes or allow it to hide its head in the crook of your arm. You can also place a towel over its head, making sure that the rabbit can still breathe. Because of its large volume-to-surface area, a rabbit can quickly overheat, so watch carefully during any procedure to make certain that the rabbit does not become overstressed. A rabbit should never be picked up by its ears because this is painful and can damage the ears. Routine veterinary care of rabbits includes nail trims, teeth checks and trims, and routine physical examinations.

To initially get control of the rabbit, scruff it just behind its ears. Grab the scruff into the palm of your hand while keeping your arm along the rabbit's body (Fig. 10-21, *A*). Reach over the rabbit to support its body by pushing it against your body and supporting its hindquarters (Fig. 10-21, *B*). It is important never to pick up a rabbit unless you have its hindquarters secure. To avoid injuring the rabbit and yourself, as previously mentioned, support its hindquarters against your body (Fig. 10-21, *C*).

FIG. 10-21

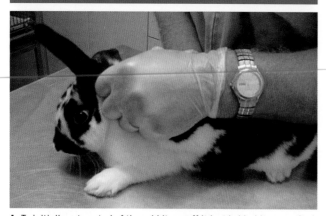

A To initially get control of the rabbit, scruff it just behind its ears. Grab the scruff into the palm of your hand while keeping your arm along the rabbit's body.

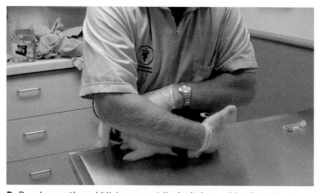

B Reach over the rabbit to support its body by pushing it against your body and supporting its hindquarters.

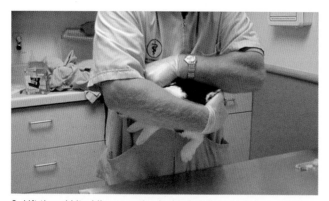

C Lift the rabbit while supporting its hindquarters against your body.

FIG. 10-22

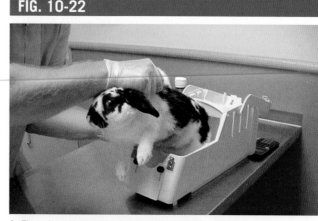

A First place the rabbit's hind end into the restrainer.

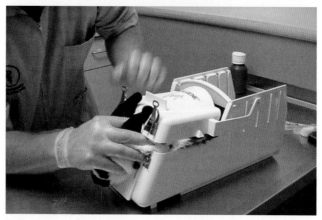

B Once the back end of the rabbit is in the restrainer, gently place its front end in and fasten the front of the restrainer.

Rabbits can be restrained in a commercial restrainer to allow safe handling of their heads. Be sure you set the restrainer before you get the rabbit out of its cage. Set the back plate so that the rabbit fits with little room to move its back end. First, place the hind end of the rabbit into the restrainer (Fig. 10-22, *A*). Once the back end of the rabbit is in the restrainer, gently place its front end in and fasten the front of the restrainer (Fig. 10-22, *B*).

To determine the sex or to examine the rabbit's urogenital area, firmly scruff the animal with your nondominant hand. On a firm surface, tip the animal back so it is sitting on its rump, supported by your body (Fig. 10-23, *A*). Examine the genital area for the lack of testicles and the presence of a vulva (Fig. 10-23, *B*). Male rabbits have testicles to either side of the genital opening. In rabbits, the inguinal rings are open so the testicles may not be in the scrotum at the time of examination. Next, check the genital opening. Gently open the genital orifice and extrude the penis.

FIG. 10-23

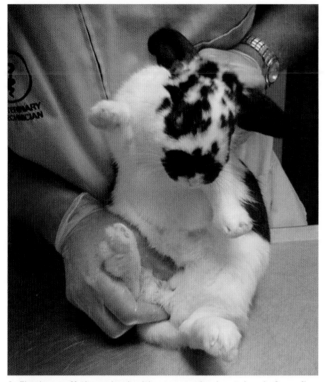

A Firmly scruff the animal with your nondominant hand. On a firm surface, tip the animal back so it is sitting on its rump, supported by your body.

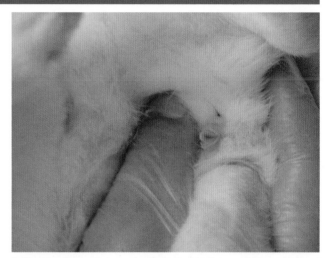

B Examine the genital area for the lack of testicles and the presence of a vulva.

INJECTIONS

Place the rabbit on a firm surface with good footing. Form a subcutaneous tent just caudal to the animal's ears. Wipe the injection area with alcohol to remove dirt and debris (Fig. 10-24, *A*). Bring the needle and syringe along the rabbit's back. If you place your hand on the rabbit's back, when the rabbit moves you will be less likely to pull the needle out as you give the injection (Fig. 10-24, *B*). Aspirate before giving the injection to ensure proper placement.

To administer an intramuscular injection, place the rabbit on a firm surface and allow it to hide in the crook of your arm. Palpate the animal's femur so that you can determine where to place the needle. Swab the injection area with alcohol (Fig. 10-25, *A*). Place the needle just caudal and parallel to the femur, being sure to aspirate before completing the injection (Fig. 10-25, *B*). An alternative site for intramuscular injection in the rabbit is the large lumbar (epaxial) muscle located along its spine. Restrain the rabbit by tucking its head under the handler's arm, palpate the site, and insert the needle at a 30-degree angle just lateral and parallel to the rabbit's spine.

FIG. 10-24

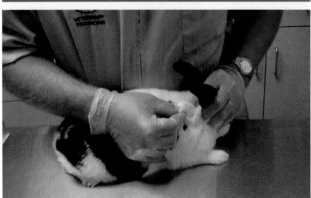

A Wipe the injection area with alcohol to remove dirt and debris.

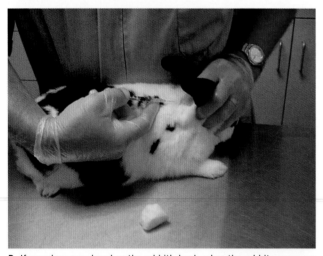

B If you place your hand on the rabbit's back, when the rabbit moves you will be less likely to pull the needle out as you give the injection.

FIG. 10-25

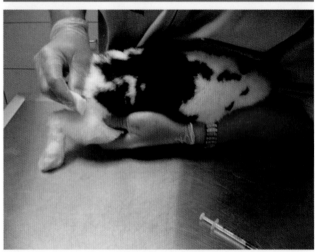

A Swab the injection area with alcohol.

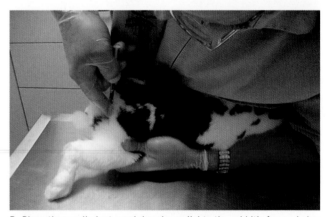

B Place the needle just caudal and parallel to the rabbit's femur, being sure to aspirate before completing the injection.

VENIPUNCTURE

You can use the marginal ear vein to obtain a small blood sample or complete an intravenous injection in the rabbit. Start by placing the rabbit safely in a restrainer or wrap it in a towel so that its back end is firmly supported. Locate its marginal ear vein, pluck the hair off it, and swab the vein with alcohol (Fig. 10-26, *A*). It is best to use a tourniquet to occlude the ear vein. The easiest method is to apply a paper clip to occlude the vessel, which allows good dilation and visualization of the vein (Fig. 10-26, *B*). Then brace the ear against your hand or a roll of gauze to give it support while you insert the needle (Fig. 10-26, *C*). When collecting a blood sample, be sure to aspirate slowly to avoid collapsing the animal's vessel. When completing an intravenous injection, remove the paper clip after ensuring needle placement before injection and inject any solutions slowly to allow the vein to clear the medication volume administered.

FIG. 10-26

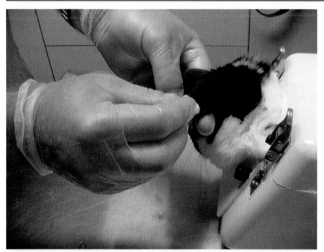

A Locate the animal's marginal ear vein, pluck the hair off it, and swab the vein with alcohol.

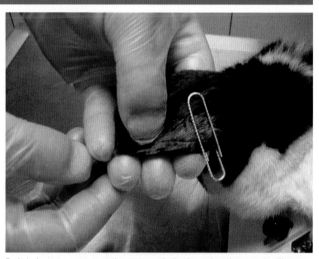

B It is best to use a tourniquet to occlude the animal's ear vein. The easiest method is to apply a paper clip to occlude the vessel, which allows good dilation and visualization of the vein.

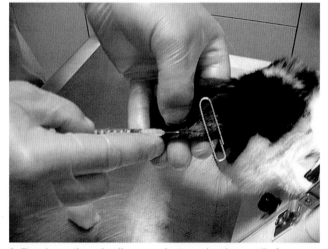

C Then brace the animal's ear against your hand or a roll of gauze to support it while you insert the needle.

THE FERRET

Ferrets are domestic animals that retain many attributes of the wild ferret. They are true carnivores and many of their behaviors can be traced to their predatory nature. The ferret's hunting instincts remain strong. Ferrets are alert and active and enjoy many new environments. Their primary means of defense is to bite, and they will resort to play biting as well as fear biting. If neutered, ferrets live companionably in groups. Instinctive behaviors remain strong in terms of territory marking as well as play behaviors. One should never underestimate a ferret's ability to maneuver into small places; its curiosity will take it into every available nook and cranny. Careful ferret proofing is necessary to prevent the animal from escaping.

When restraining a ferret, it is always important to have good control of its head. Ferrets are very flexible and can twist almost 180 degrees. Maintain good head control by placing your index finger on one side of the animal's mandible with your middle finger on the other (Fig. 10-27, *A*). Be sure to keep the ferret's body along your arm for support. You can then place your thumb and ring finger around the ferret's front limbs and support it by its armpits (Fig. 10-27, *B*). In addition, ferrets are curious and easily distracted, so placing a palatable paste or ferret supplement drops on the animal's abdomen for it to lick off will often occupy a ferret long enough for many short procedures such as nail trims, ear examinations, or quick physical examinations (Fig. 10-27, *C* and *D*). If you are working with a ferret and need to settle it down

FIG. 10-27

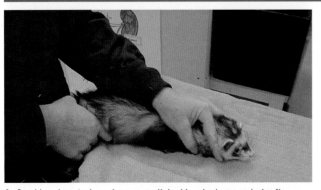

A Good head control can be accomplished by placing your index finger on one side of the mandible with your middle finger on the other.

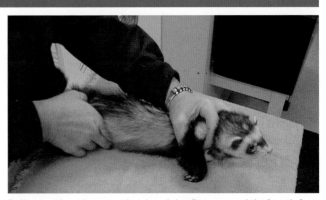

B You can then place your thumb and ring finger around the ferret's front limbs and support it by its armpits.

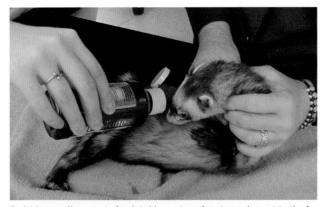

C Add a small amount of palatable paste or ferret supplement to the fur on the animal's ventral abdomen.

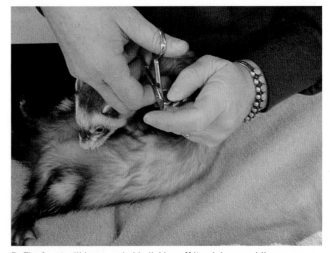

D The ferret will be occupied in licking off its abdomen while you accomplish the needed procedure.

or simply want your hands free for a short period, most ferrets are very happy in your pocket (Fig. 10-28).

When physical restraint is necessary, scruffing the ferret and holding it along your arm works well. Be sure you grab enough scruff into the palm of your hand and scruff high on the animal's neck near the ears (Fig. 10-29, *A*). To prevent the ferret from twisting and to better support the animal, hold it against your arm (Fig. 10-29, *B*). If you need to deal with the ferret's head, placing the animal in a towel works as a good method of restraint. First, lay the towel out flat on the table, then place the ferret in the middle and wrap the towel tightly over the ferret, tucking one side under the other. Be sure to keep the towel snug around the animal's neck so the ferret cannot escape (Fig. 10-29, *C*).

Ear cleaning is a common procedure that must be performed in the ferret. Simply scruff the ferret and keep it close to your body (Fig. 10-30). Ferrets can be trained to allow ear cleaning as a matter of routine health care.

INJECTIONS

To administer a subcutaneous injection, scruff the ferret and wipe the injection site off with alcohol. Be sure the ferret has good footing and hold it firmly to your body with your arm (Fig. 10-31, *A*). Bring the injection needle into the tented scruff while holding the animal close to your body so that if the ferret suddenly moves it will not pull out the needle (Fig. 10-31, *B*). Aspirate before completing the injection.

FIG. 10-28

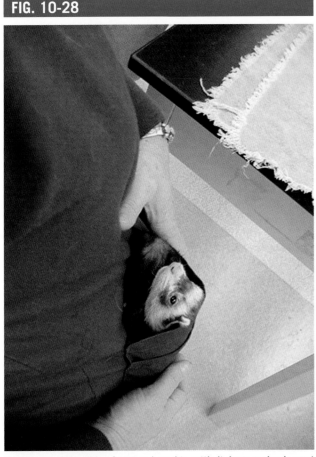

If you are working with a ferret and need to settle it down or simply want your hands free for a short period, most ferrets are very happy in your pocket.

FIG. 10-29

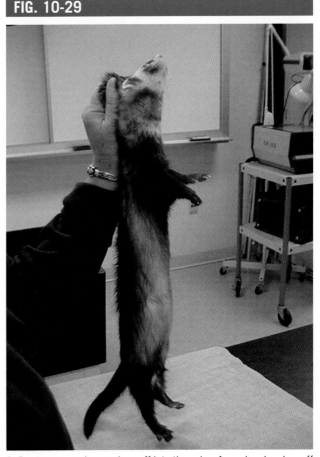

A Be sure you grab enough scruff into the palm of your hand and scruff high on the ferret's neck near its ears.

(Figure 10-29, continued on following page)

FIG. 10-29 cont.

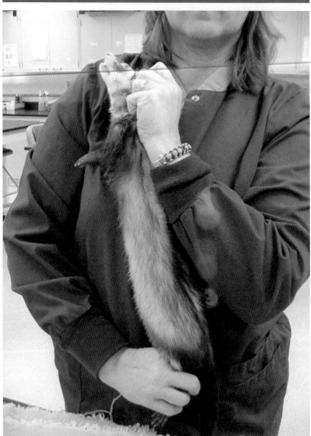

B To prevent the ferret from twisting and to better support the animal hold the animal against your arm for support.

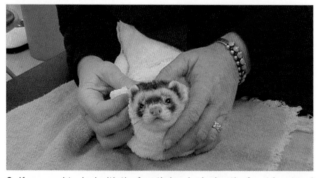

C If you need to deal with the ferret's head, placing the ferret in a towel works as a good method of restraint.

FIG. 10-30

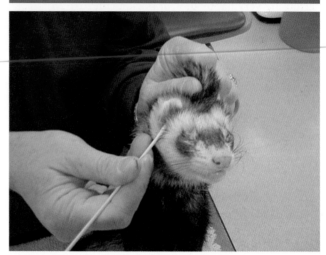

Simply scruff the ferret and keep it close to your body.

FIG. 10-31

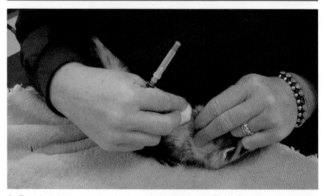

A To administer a subcutaneous injection, scruff the ferret and wipe the injection site off with alcohol.

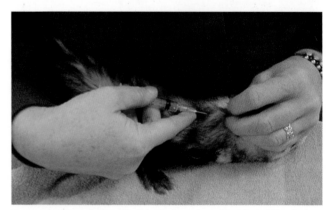

B Bring the injection needle into the tented scruff while holding it close to the body so that if the ferret suddenly moves it will not pull out the needle.

To complete an intramuscular injection in the muscles of the ferret's caudal thigh, scruff the ferret and hold its body firmly along your arm (Fig. 10-32, *A*). Intramuscular injections require two people: one person to restrain the animal and the other person to perform the injection. Locate the animal's femur by palpation. Once you locate the femur, place your thumb over the top of it, isolating the ferret's caudal thigh. Place the needle in the animal's caudal thigh at a 45-degree angle, aspirate, and complete the injection (Fig. 10-32, *B*). An alternative, if you have a wiggly ferret, is to place it in a scruff hold while supporting its body along your arm, as described earlier, then have someone place a towel over the ferret's head (Fig. 10-32, *C*). This will often distract the ferret long enough to complete the procedure.

BLOOD COLLECTION

You can collect blood from the ferret's jugular vein. Restrain the ferret as you would a cat. Draping the ferret's legs over the table edge exposes the jugular vein. To expose the left jugular vein, hold the ferret's head with your right hand, keeping your right arm tight over its body so that you hold the animal close to your body. Drape its front legs over the edge of the table with your left hand (Fig. 10-33, *A*). To expose the right jugular vein, hold the animal's head with your left hand and the ferret's body close to your body with your left arm. Be sure to use your outside arm to hold the animal's head and your outside arm to pin the ferret's body to your body to prevent twisting. Drape the ferret's legs over the edge of the

FIG. 10-32

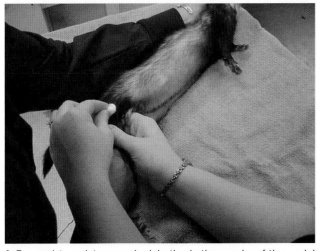

A To complete an intramuscular injection in the muscles of the caudal thigh, scruff the ferret and hold its body firmly along your arm.

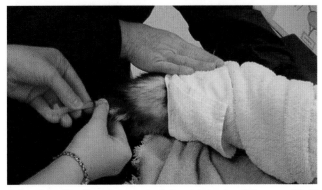

C An alternative, if you have a wiggly ferret, is to place it in a scruff hold with its body supported along your arm as previously described, then have someone place a towel over the ferret's head.

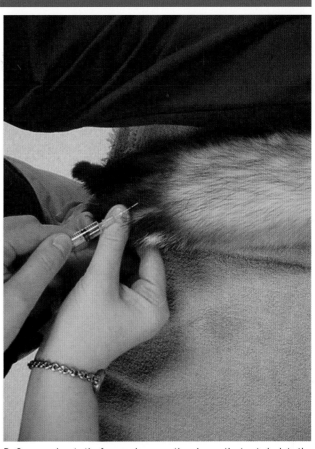

B Once you locate the femur, place your thumb over the top to isolate the caudal thigh. Place the needle in the caudal thigh at a 45-degree angle, aspirate, and complete the injection.

FIG. 10-33

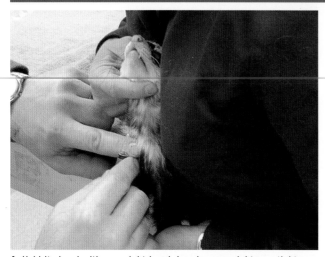

A Hold its head with your right hand, keeping your right arm tight over the ferret's body so that the animal is close to your body.

B Be sure to use your outside arm to hold the ferret's head and your outside arm to pin the ferret's body to your body to prevent twisting.

table with your right hand. To distract the ferret, you can talk to it, blow on its nose, or shake its head gently. An alternative method of restraint for a jugular venipuncture is to hold the ferret in lateral recumbency. You will need to hyperextend your wrist to adequately expose the vein (Fig. 10-33, *B*).

SUGGESTED READINGS

Beynon PH, Cooper JE: *Manual of exotic pets*, Gloucestershire, 1991, British Small Animal Veterinary Association.

Coria-Avila GA, Gavrila AM, Ménard S, Ismail N, Pfaus JG: Cecum location in rats and the implications for intraperitoneal injections, *Lab Anim* 36(7):25–30, 2007.

Fowler ME: *Restraint and handling of wild and domestic animals*, Ames, IA, 1978, Iowa State University Press.

Lawson PT: *ALAT training manual*, Memphis, 1999, Sheridan.

Sonsthagen TF: *Restraint of domestic animals*, St. Louis, 1991, Mosby.

Svendsen P, Hau J: *Handbook of laboratory animal science* (vol 1), Ann Arbor, 1994, CRC Press.

Todd-Jenkins K, Dugan B, Remsburg DW, Montgomery C: Restraint and handling of animals. In *McCurnin's clinical textbook for veterinary technicians*, ed 8, Philadelphia, 2014, Saunders.

11

Restraint of Birds

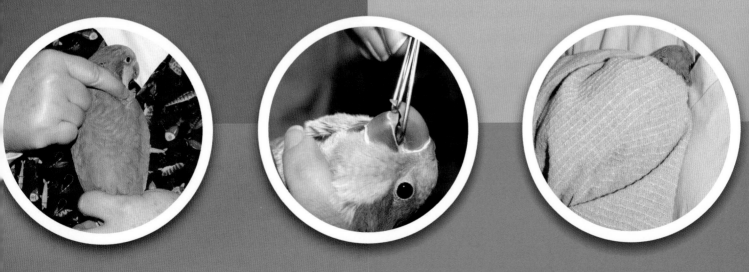

Caged birds, such as parakeets, canaries, finches, parrots, cockatiels, and pigeons, are being seen more in veterinary practices than ever before. Many clients who live in an apartment building that may not allow dogs or cats have found these pets to be perfect. Unfortunately, birds are highly sensitive to stress and rough handling, which can cause broken wings or legs, progression of a disease process, and even death. Owners often do not know how to properly care for or feed their feathered friends, so trips to the veterinary hospital may occur quite frequently.

Birds can defend themselves with their beaks. The larger birds can readily mangle a finger or easily take a fingertip off. They also have sharp toenails, and larger birds can injure you with their wings. Domestic fowl have the same weapons, and the legs of a rooster have spurs that can cause quite a septic wound if the rooster scratches someone. It takes practice and patience to work with these animals successfully and safely. As with other species, you must use the least restraint necessary to get the job done.

TRANSPORT TO CLINIC

Advise the client to bring the bird in its own cage if possible. The client should remove all the toys, food, and water dishes and all but one perch to make the trip. If the dishes fill holes that the bird can escape from, the client should empty the dishes and put them back in the slots. This keeps the bird from injuring itself if it falls off the perch during transport. Ask the client to keep the droppings tray, with papers in place, in the cage. Droppings can reveal a lot about the bird's health, so you will want to examine droppings from the last 12 to 24 hours. If the cage is too large to bring in, ask clients to bring the dropping papers with them. The client can easily fold up the paper and put it into a grocery bag for transport.

If the weather is cold, the client should get the interior of the car warm and place a blanket over the bird's cage. The blanket helps to keep drafts from the bird and will make it feel more secure. During hot weather, the bird should not be positioned in front of the air conditioning vent. Drafts will make a sick bird sicker.

CAPTURING THE BIRD

SMALL BIRDS

Most tame birds have been trained to hop onto a person's finger or hand, after which the veterinary professional can easily grasp them from behind. However, if you are not fast enough, the bird may fly off your hand and escape into the examination room. Capturing small to medium-sized birds in a cage prevents accidental escape into the examination room and is the preferred method of capture. Open the cage door and remove the perch and dishes. This makes the bird sit on the floor of the cage or hang onto the bars. Reach in with a lightweight towel, like a sackcloth or a thin terrycloth towel, and grasp the bird from behind, trying to get its head between your thumb and index finger (Fig. 11-1, A). Be *very* careful not to squeeze the bird's chest and abdomen because you can easily suffocate a bird with even slight pressure. Bring the bird out of the cage and put the front of the bird up against your chest (Fig. 11-1, B). Find the bird's head and reposition your thumb and index finger under its jaw and around its throat, or you can hold it by the sides of its head (Fig. 11-1, C). Note that in the figure the towel has been removed so you can see what is going on; usually you will work through the towel. Be careful not to place your fingers over the bird's eyes, as you can damage them. If one hand is too small to hold a medium-sized bird, you can use your other hand to grasp the bird's feet and wing tips. Your other fingers should be held either straight out away from the body or curled in without touching the body (Fig. 11-1, D). If you wrap your other fingers around the bird's body, you could suffocate the bird by applying too

FIG. 11-1

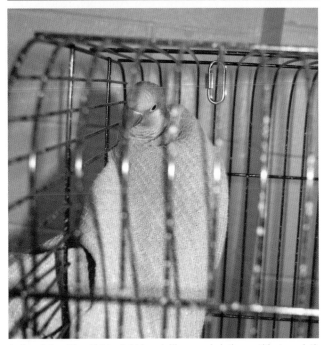

A Reach in with a lightweight towel, like a sackcloth or a thin terrycloth towel, and grasp the bird from behind, trying to get its head between your thumb and index finger.

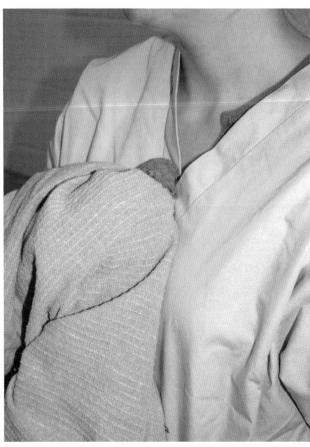

B Bring the bird out of the cage and put the front of the bird up against your chest.

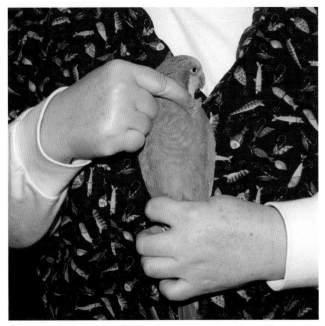

C Find the bird's head and reposition your thumb and index finger under its jaw and around its throat or you can hold it by the sides of its head.

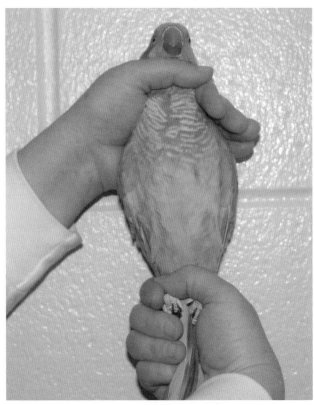

D Your other fingers should be either straight out away from the bird's body or curled in without touching the body.

much pressure to its thorax and abdomen. For small birds like parakeets, use your little finger to pin its legs and wing tips to the palm of your hand (Fig. 11-2). You can now discard the towel or you can choose to work through the towel, which many veterinary professionals prefer to do. You can use the towel to cover the bird's eyes, which not only will help to calm the bird but will give it something to chew on, thereby keeping its beak busy (Fig. 11-3).

FIG. 11-2

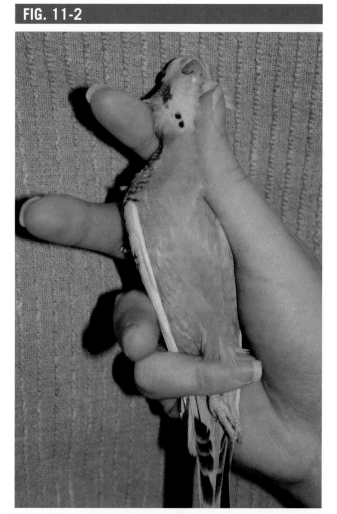

For small birds such as parakeets, use your little finger to pin the bird's legs and wing tips to the palm of your hand.

LARGE BIRDS

Large birds such as macaws and Amazons require two hands and a thicker towel or gauntlets. If the bird is in a cage that has a door big enough to reach through and bring it out, then capture it in the cage. This prevents the bird from escaping and being free in the examination room. However, a large bird is usually brought into the clinic in a carrier. You simply place the carrier on the floor, take the lid off and allow the bird to walk out, which most birds readily do. In either case, come up from behind the bird and quickly and decisively encircle its neck with your index finger and thumb, making sure you get very close to the bottom of its lower beak or on either side of its head (Fig. 11-4, *A*); at the same time use your other hand to encircle its feet and wing tips. Move the bird to an examination table that has been cushioned with a couple of layers of padding. Lay your forearm down on the table with the bird's head resting in your hand. Slide your other hand around so that you are holding the bird's legs (Fig. 11-4, *B*).

FIG. 11-3

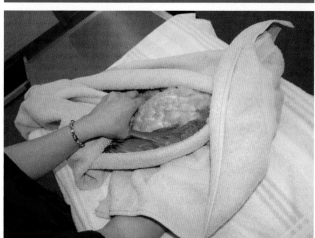

Use the towel to cover the bird's eyes; this not only will calm the bird but will give it something to chew on, thereby keeping its beak busy.

If you are wearing gloves, now is the time to take them off. Wrap the bird's feet in a towel and hold the bird's head with one hand while you shake the glove off the other hand. Then reverse hands, holding the bird's head with the ungloved hand while shaking off the remaining glove. When working with raptors, never take off your gloves! As mentioned previously, a large bird can mangle if not nip off a fingertip. Large birds can also cause severe wounds to skin because they tend to grind it between their beaks.

One drawback of gloves is that they greatly reduce tactile feeling, resulting in damage to the bird, so when you have to work on a bird with your gloves on, constantly monitor how the bird is doing. Your experience will determine whether you work with or without gloves.

If you happen to be in a large aviary or the bird has escaped, use a fine fishing net to scoop the bird out of the air or tree limb. Once the bird is in the net, quickly pin the net down to the floor and grasp the bird's head and feet. The tricky part is getting the bird out of the netting without getting tangled up.

Passerines, seed-eating birds, are fairly easy to restrain. Capture them the same way as described for the small to medium-sized parrots, but instead of holding the bird's head between your thumb and index finger hold the bird between your index and middle finger (Fig. 11-4, *C*). Hold the bird's tail and feet as previously described for parrots.

FIG. 11-4

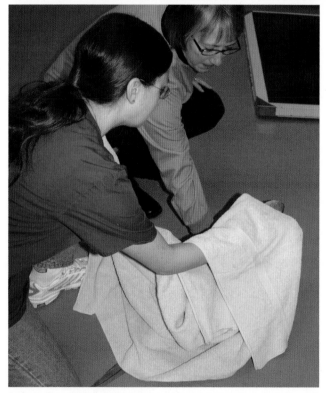

A Come from behind the bird and quickly and decisively encircle its neck with your index finger and thumb, making sure you get very close to the bottom of its lower beak or on either side of its head; at the same time, use your other hand to encircle the bird's feet and wing tips.

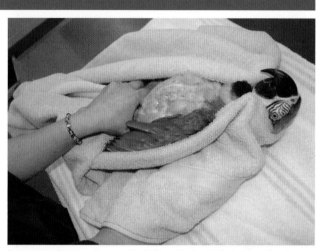

B Lay your forearm down on the table with the bird's head resting in your hand. Slide your other hand around so that you are holding the bird's legs.

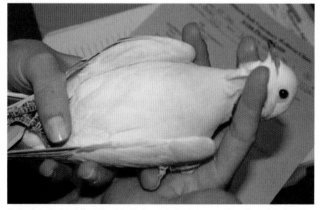

C Instead of holding the bird's head between your thumb and index finger, hold it between your index and middle finger.

You can usually catch a domestic fowl by grasping it by the leg and hanging it upside down until you are ready to treat it. These birds do flap their wings and get quite agitated, so hold them away from your body. When you are ready to examine the bird, bring its other leg up to the same hand you are using to hold the first leg. Swing the bird's body up and cradle it between your arm and body with your other arm while retaining control of its feet. Grasp the bird around the neck with your other hand. Be careful not to squeeze the bird's body; hold it fairly loosely so that you do not hinder the bird's breathing or rupture its air sac.

Take care not to squeeze a bird's thorax, abdomen, or crop when restraining it. Too much pressure to the thorax prevents the bird's lungs from inflating. Too much pressure to the abdomen may cause the bird's air sac(s) to rupture. Too much pressure on the crop can cause the bird to regurgitate, especially youngsters that have just been fed.

You will perform most procedures while holding the bird as you captured it. Once you have completed the procedure, return the bird to its cage. Gently set it on the floor, making sure that it regains its feet before you let go; then remove your hand. Do not set the bird on a perch because it could be a bit dazed and may fall off, possibly injuring itself. Once the bird has its bearings, it will hop up onto the perch.

RESTRAINT FOR MEDICAL PROCEDURES

ORAL MEDICATIONS

Liquid medications are given with the bird's head elevated above the horizontal plane to prevent aspiration. Hold the bird's head and body as previously described. If you are going to pass a tube into the bird's stomach, hold open its beak so the bird does not bite through the tube.

A paper clip works well as a speculum for small to medium-sized birds, but use manufactured specula for the large birds. To apply the paper clip speculum, tilt the paper clip slightly to one side and place the bird's upper beak in the short inside loop of the clip (Fig. 11-5, *A*). Then swing the clip down and place the end inside the bird's lower beak by pulling up on its upper beak with the clip (Fig. 11-5, *B*). Use different-sized clips for different-sized birds (Fig. 11-5, *C*). You can also use this or a speculum when you need to swab the bird's mouth or throat.

Dosing needles can also be used to deliver oral medications. Hold the bird as previously described; bring the dosing needle up to the bird's mouth and use it to push the bird's beak open. Slide the dosing needle along the bird's hard pallet and visualize it going down the esophagus.

FIG. 11-5

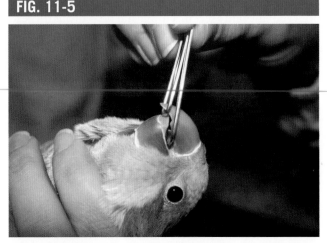

A To apply the paper clip speculum, tilt the paper clip slightly to one side and place the bird's upper beak in the short inside loop of the clip.

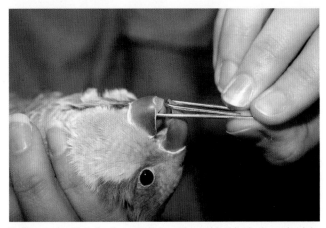

B Then swing the clip down and place the end inside the lower beak by pulling up on the upper beak up with the clip.

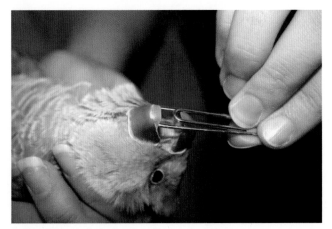

C Use different-sized clips for different sized birds.

FIG. 11-6

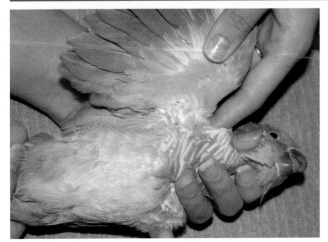

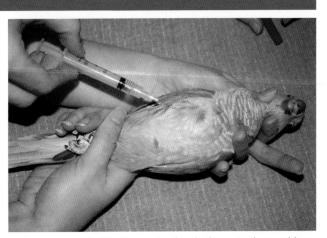

A The person giving the injection will slowly stretch one wing out to expose the axillary region.

B The intramuscular injection can be given in the pectoral or quadriceps muscle.

INJECTIONS

Injections can be given by subcutaneous or intramuscular routes. To give a subcutaneous injection, hold the bird as previously described. Lay the bird down on a padded surface as described for the large birds. The person giving the injection will slowly stretch one wing out to expose the axillary region (Fig. 11-6, *A*). For the subcutaneous injection, grasp the bird's loose skin and gently tent it. Give the intramuscular injection in the bird's pectoral or quadriceps muscle (Fig. 11-6, *B*).

VENIPUNCTURE

Venipuncture can be done on the right jugular vein or the brachial vein located in the wing. For jugular venipuncture, hold the bird as described for the large birds. Slightly tilt the bird so its right jugular is topmost to the person doing the venipuncture. Use your thumb to hold back the bird's feathers and occlude the vein (Fig. 11-7). Do not extend the bird's neck too far to the left, as this can kink the trachea and cause suffocation. Expose the brachial vein using the same hold as described for the subcutaneous injection.

FIG. 11-7

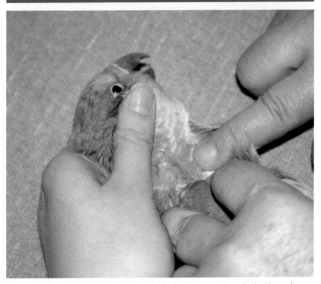

Use your thumb to hold back the bird's feathers and occlude the vein.

FIG. 11-8

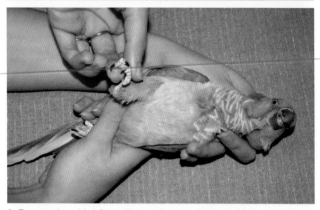

A To restrain a bird for splint application, hold the bird as previously described for large birds. This hold allows the restrainer to tilt the bird to the left or right to present the left or right wing or leg.

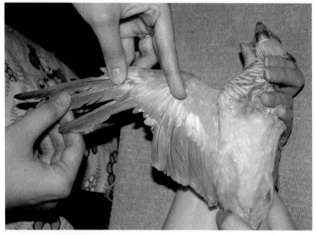

B Most of the time it is easier on both the bird and you if someone else performs this task.

SPLINT APPLICATION

Fractured wings and legs are often treated by the application of tape splints. To restrain a bird for splint application, hold the bird as previously described for large birds. This hold allows the restrainer to tilt the bird to the left or right to present the left or right wing or leg (Fig. 11-8, *A*). If the bird is small enough, you may be able to hold it in one hand and help hold the wing or leg. However, most of the time it is easier on both the bird and you if someone else performs this task (Fig. 11-8, *B*).

FIG. 11-9

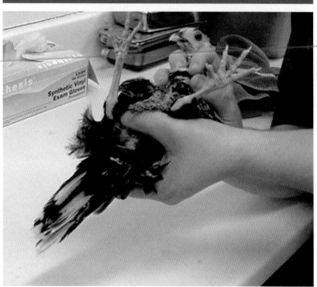

Tilt the bird so that its rear is up slightly, let go of its legs, and allow them to curl up toward the bird's chest. Hang on to the bird's tail, if present, to expose the cloacal opening.

CLOACAL SWAB

A common diagnostic test on birds is to swab the cloacae. The cloacae is the common opening of the urogenital tract. To accomplish this test, tilt the bird so that its rear is up slightly, let go of the legs, and allow them to curl up toward the chest. Hang on to the bird's tail, if present, to expose the cloacal opening (Fig. 11-9).

FIG. 11-10

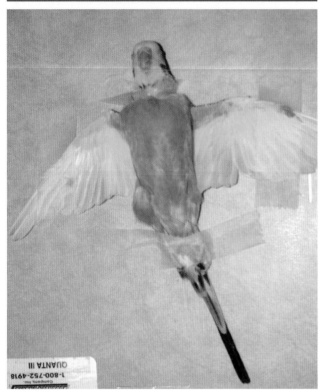

In restraining birds for radiographic procedures, all birds should be anesthetized if possible. Small to medium-sized birds can be taped directly to the cassette with paper tape.

RADIOGRAPHY

In restraining birds for radiographic procedures, all birds should be anesthetized if possible. Small to medium-sized birds can be taped directly to the cassette with paper tape (Fig. 11-10). You may need to use tape, gauze bandages, and radiographic weights to hold large birds in position. Remember that your hands and fingers should never be in the primary beam. There are specially designed boards to restrain birds for radiographs and these boards should be a part of your inventory if you treat a large number of birds.

ELIZABETHAN COLLAR

An Elizabethan collar is often necessary to prevent a bird from picking at its bandages or a wound. You can use various materials to fashion collars, including playing cards, plastic detergent bottles, pieces of cardboard, and pieces of x-ray film. These work well for smaller birds. For larger birds, you will need to fashion the collar out of thick leather or sturdy plastic. All birds will destroy an Elizabethan collar if they can chew on it.

BEAK RESTRAINT

If the bird is a ferocious biter, you can place a mouth speculum to keep the beak wedged open. If its beak is long and pointed like a turkey or some of the wading birds, you can place a cork on the end of it. This prevents the bird from plucking your eyeball out, but this precaution will not prevent the bird from giving you a pretty good black eye if it should strike. Therefore you should never let go of the bird's neck/head until you have completed all procedures and you can safely set the bird down and move out of the way. Also be careful when removing the speculum, cork, or tape because the bird may retaliate by biting. Eye protection is a must when working with these types of birds.

SUGGESTED READINGS

Burr EW: *Companion bird medicine*, Ames, IA, 1987, Iowa State University Press.

DeLong G, Okumura S: *Nursing care of cage birds, reptiles, and amphibians: principles and practices of veterinary technician*, St. Louis, 2004, Mosby.

Fowler ME: *Restraint and handling of wild and domestic animals*, Ames, IA, 1978, Iowa State University Press.

Petrak ML: *Diseases of cage and aviary birds*, ed 2, Philadelphia, 1982, Lea & Febiger.

Sonsthagen TF: *Restraint of domestic animals*, St. Louis, 1991, Mosby.

Steiner, Davis: *Caged bird medicine*, Ames, IA, 1981, Iowa State University Press.

Gender Names

DOG

Male: Dog or Stud
Female: Bitch
Newborn/young: Pup

CAT

Male: Tom
Female: Queen
Newborn/young: Kitten

HORSE

Male: Stallion or Stud
Female: Mare
Young male: Colt
Young female: Filly
Newborn (either sex): Foal
Castrated male: Gelding

CATTLE

Male: Bull
Female: Cow
Young male: Bullock, bull calf
Young female: Heifer
Newborn: Calf
Castrated male: Steer

PIG

Male: Boar
Female: Sow
Young female: Gilt
Young male, uncastrated: Boar pig
Male castrated before maturity: Barrow
Male castrated after maturity: Stag
Young of either sex: Shoat
Newborn: Piglet

SHEEP

Male: Ram or Buck
Female: Ewe
Newborn/young: Lamb
Castrated male: Wether

GOAT

Male: Billy or Buck
Female: Nanny or Doe
Newborn/young: Kid
Castrated male: Wether

RABBIT

Male: Buck
Female: Doe
Newborn/young: Kit

FERRET

Male: Hob
Female: Jill
Newborn/young: Kit

SUGGESTED READINGS

Hrapkiewiczs K, Medina L, Holmes DD: *Clinical laboratory animal medicine*, Ames, IA, 1998, Iowa State University Press.
Sonsthagen TF: *Restraint of domestic animals*, St. Louis, 1991, Mosby.
Taylor RE, Field TG: *Scientific farm animal production*, Upper Saddle River, NJ, 2016, Prentice Hall.

Physiologic Data

Species	Rectal Temperature (°F)	Pulse Rate (beats/min)	Respiratory Rate (breaths/min)
Dog	100.0-102.5	70-180	10-30
Cat	100.5-102.5	110-130	20-30
Horse	99.5-101.3	28-50	8-16
Cattle	100.5-103	40-70	10-30
Swine	100-104	58-100	8-18
Sheep	102-104	60-90	12-19
Goat	102-104	60-90	12-19
Rabbit	101.3-104	130-325	30-60
Ferret	100-104	200-400	33-36
Mice	97.5-100.4	325-780	60-220
Rat	96.6-99.5	250-450	70-115
Hamster	98.6-100.4	250-500	35-135
Gerbil	98.6-101.3	360	70-120
Guinea pig	99-103.1	230-380	42-104

From Sonsthagen TF: *Restraint of domestic animals*, St. Louis, 1991, Mosby; and Hrapkiewicz K, Medina L, Holmes D: *Clinical laboratory animal medicine*, Ames, IA, 1998, Iowa State University Press.

GLOSSARY

A

Aggressive: A fighting disposition

Anesthesia: Loss of sensation with or without loss of consciousness

Bight: A sharp bend in a rope

B

Bolus: Medication delivered in one large dose or a preparation of oral medication given to large animals

Bovine: Of or relating to oxen or cattle

Brachycephalic: Referring to short-nosed breeds of dogs, such as the boxer, English bulldog, and pug

Butt: To thrust or push with the head or horns

C

Calving: The act of a cow's giving birth

Canine: Of or relating to dogs

Caprine: Of or relating to goats

Cast: To throw to the ground, usually with a variety of ropes and knots

Caudal: Situated in or directed toward the hind part of the body

Cephalic vein: A blood vessel located in the cranial aspect of the front leg

Cervical vertebrae: Spinal bones in the neck

Chute: A capture device made of metal or wood that restrains cattle

Coccygeal vertebrae: Spinal bones of the tail

Commissure: Junction between two parts, such as the lips or eyelids

Constructive tonalities: Using the voice in a commanding way

Corral: Pen or enclosure for confining or capturing livestock

Cranial: Situated in or directed toward the front part of the body

D

Distal: Away from the point of attachment or axis of the body

Distraction technique: The use of mild pain to distract the attention of an animal so a procedure can be performed

Dock: The part of an animal's tail left after amputation

Dorsal: Toward the spine or upper side of the body

Drench: A large dose of medicine mixed with liquid and given down the throat of an animal

E

End: The end of a rope that can be freely moved about when tying a knot

F

Far side: The right side of a horse

Farrow: The act of a sow's giving birth

Feline: Of or relating to cats

Femoral vein: Located on the medial side of the hind leg, between the sartorius and gracilis muscles

Fetlock: The leg joint above the hoof of a horse or other hooved animal

Flank: Laying an animal on its side

Foaling: The act of a mare's giving birth

Friable: Easily broken or pulverized

G

Gauntlets: Heavy leather gloves used to restrain animals

Gurney: A wheeled cot or stretcher

H

Half hitch: A complete circle formed in a rope when making a knot or hitch

Head shy: Wariness of having the head approached or touched

Hematoma: Swelling or a mass of blood confined to an organ, tissue, or space, caused by a break in a blood vessel

Herbivore: A plant-eating animal

Hitch: A temporary fastening of a rope to a hook, post, or other object with the rope arranged so the standing part forces the end against the object with sufficient pressure to prevent slipping

Hobble: A device used to fasten together the legs of an animal to prevent straying or kicking

Hock: The tarsal joint or region in the hind limb of animals that corresponds to the ankle in people

Hurdle: A portable panel used to herd livestock

Hyperthermia: Abnormally high body temperature

Hypothermia: Abnormally low body temperature

Hypoxia: A deficiency of oxygen reaching the tissues of the body

J

Jugular veins: Paired major blood vessels running lateral to the trachea

K

Kindling: The act of a female rabbit's giving birth

Knot: Intertwining of one or two ropes in which the pressure of the standing part of the rope alone prevents the end from slipping

L

Lambing: The act of a ewe's giving birth

Lateral: Situated in or directed toward the side of the body, away from the body axis

Lateral recumbency: Reclining on the side of the body

Lateral saphenous vein: A blood vessel on the lateral aspect of the leg just distal to the hock

Lavage: Washing out of a cavity

Lumbar vertebrae: Spinal bones between the chest and pelvis

M

Mandible: The lower jaw

Medial: Situated in or directed toward the axis of the body

Metatarsus: Part of the hind foot in quadrupeds, distal to the tarsus or ankle

Muzzle: A covering for an animal's mouth to prevent eating or biting

N

Near side: The left side of a horse

O

Obese: Excessively fat

Occluding: Closing or holding off, such as occluding a vessel for venipuncture

Off side: The right side of a horse

Overhand knot: A basic knot used in more complex knots

Ovine: Of or relating to sheep

P

Palpation: To examine by touch

Per os: By mouth

Pinch biting: Biting with the incisors by a muzzled dog or cat

Pinna: Ear flap

Porcine: Of or relating to pigs

Proximal: Toward the point of attachment or axis of the body

Q

Queening: The act of a female cat's giving birth

R

Restraint: Forceful prevention of movement or activity by physical or chemical means

S

Stanchion: A device that fits loosely around a cow's neck and limits forward and backward motion

Standing part: The longer end of the rope that is attached to the animal

Stocks: A small, square restraining pen with a front and back gate

T

Territory: Area, such as a nesting or denning site and foraging range, defended by an animal or group of animals

Thoracic vertebrae: Spinal bones of the chest area

Throw: The wrapping of one rope around another to make a knot

Twitch: Chain, rope, or strap that is tightened over a horse's lip as a restraining device

V

Venipuncture: Puncture of a vein for withdrawal of blood or injection

Venipuncturist: One who performs a venipuncture

Ventral: Away from the spine or upper side of the body

W

Whelping: The act of a bitch's giving birth

Withers: The area between the shoulder blades of a horse

Note: Page numbers followed by *f* indicate figures, and *t* indicate tables.

A

Aggression, signs of, 108
Aggressive dogs, 57, 62–64, 62*f*, 64*f*
Animal safety, 3–4
Animals
  herd, horses as, 132
  pigs can be vicious, 178
  prey (cattle), 108
  restraint on, 2
  sick or injured, 3
  some are extremely territorial, 3
  unrestrained large, 3
Antikicking devices (cattle), 126, 126*f*
Application
  splint, in birds, 226, 226*f*
  tourniquet (dogs), 93, 93*f*
Approaching horses, 134–138, 135*f*, 137–138*f*
Aspirate, for mouse, 194
Auscultation, in restrained horses, 133*f*

B

Bags
  nylon or canvas, 48
  restraint (cats), 48–50, 48*f*, 50*f*
Barriers (pigs), 178–179
Battering rams, 3
Beak restraint, 227
Beaks to peck or pinch with, 3
Behavior, of cats, 24
Bend, sheet, 16, 16*f*
Bight, 8, 8*f*
  bowline on, 18, 18*f*
Birds
  caged, 220
  capturing, 220–224
  large, 222–224, 222–223*f*
  restraint of, 219–227
    for medical procedures, 224–227
    transport to clinic, 220
  small, 220–222, 221–222*f*
  stress in, 220
Bitches, pregnant, 57
Biting, as means of communication,
    in horses, 132
Blankets, 103, 103*f*
  cats, 47, 47*f*
Blindfolds, for horses, 143, 143*f*
Blood, drawing of, in restrained horses, 133*f*
Blood collection
  ferret for, 217–218, 218*f*
  rat for, 200, 200*f*
Boars, 3
Body language
  of animals, 4
  of cats, 24
  of horses, 132
Bow knot
  double, 12, 13*f*
  single, 12, 12*f*

Bowline
  on bight, 18, 18*f*
  knot, 16–17, 17*f*
Buckets (pigs), 179
Bulls, 3
  unpredictability of, 108

C

Cage retrieval and restraint (mouse), 188, 189*f*
Caged birds, 220
Caged dogs, handling, 58–64, 58*f*
  aggressive dogs, 62–64, 62*f*, 64*f*
  calm dogs, 59–60, 59*f*, 61*f*
  large friendly dogs, 59–60, 59*f*, 61*f*
  nervous dogs, 62–64, 62*f*, 64*f*
Cages or carrier
  removing from (cats), 27–29, 27*f*, 29*f*
  returning to (cats), 30, 30*f*
Calm dogs, 59–60, 59*f*, 61*f*
Calming, of horses, 132
Calves
  placing in lateral recumbency, 128, 129*f*
  restraint of, 128
    flanking of, 128, 129*f*
  separating from cow, 110
Canine teeth, dog's, 56
Canvas bags, nylon or (cats), 48
Capture
  of goat, 170
  of kid, 175
Capture poles (dogs), 102, 102*f*
Capturing
  bird, 220–224
  horses, 134–138, 135*f*, 137*f*
  pigs, 178–179
  sheep, 160, 160*f*
Carriers
  removing from cages or (cats), 27–29, 27*f*, 29*f*
  returning to cages or (cats), 30, 30*f*
Carrying
  cats, 31, 31*f*
  dogs, 68–72
  dogs weighing more than 50 lbs, 72, 72*f*
  5- to 50-lb dogs, 68–71, 68*f*, 70–71*f*
  or lifting pigs, 180, 181*f*
Castration
  restraint for (lambs), 167
  restraint for dehorning and (goats), 175
Cats
  behavior of, 24
  body language of, 24
  carrying, 31, 31*f*
  dominance over, 24
  gender names, 229
  guidelines for restraining, 25–31
    carrying a cat, 31, 31*f*
    removing a collar, 26, 26*f*
    removing from cage or carrier, 27–30,
      27*f*, 29–30*f*

Cats (*Continued*)
    restraining heads, 25, 25*f*
    restraining legs, 26, 26*f*
  lassos, 52, 52*f*
  muzzles, 50, 51*f*
  physiologic data of, 231*t*
  precautions for restraining, 24–25
  restraint bags, 48–50, 48*f*, 50*f*
  restraint of, 23–53
    applying tourniquets for cephalic
      venipunctures, 41–43, 41–43*f*
    behavior of, 24
    equipment for, 44–52
    guidelines for, 25–31
    for nail trimming, 44, 44*f*
    precautions for restraining cats, 24–25
    techniques for, 32–38
    for venipunctures, 39, 40*f*
  retain instinctive behavior as predators, 24
Cat's left side will touch table, 35, 36*f*
Cat's right side will touch table, 37, 37*f*
Cattle
  and dogs, 110
  gender names, 229
  getting away from threatening
    situation of, 108
  herding of, 108–110, 108*f*, 110*f*
  kicking of, 108
  means of defense, 108
  physiologic data of, 231*t*
  restraint of, 107–130
    antikicking devices for, 126, 126*f*
    of calves, 128
    in chutes and stanchions, 111–114,
      111*f*, 114*f*
    of head, 116–120
    lifting legs in, 123–124, 123–124*f*
    oral medications for, 122, 122*f*
    using tail, 126–127
Caveman pats, for horses, 143
Cephalic veins (goats), 173
Cephalic venipuncture
  applying tourniquets for (cats), 41–43, 41–43*f*
  dogs, 91, 91*f*
Chain, neck (goats), 172
Chain shank, for horses, 149, 149*f*
Chain twitch, for horses, 145, 145–146*f*
Chamber, inhalation, cats, 52
Chemical restraint, 3, 5
  cats, 52, 52*f*
Chutes
  many types of (cattle), 114
  and stanchions, restraint in (cattle),
    111–114, 111*f*, 114*f*
Claws, of domestic animals, 3
Cleaning, ear, in ferret, 215
Clients, not having them restrain their dogs, 56
Clinic, transport to, in restraint of birds, 220
Cloacal swab, in birds, 226, 226*f*

Clove hitch, 21, 21*f*
Collars
    Elizabethan, in birds, 227
    goats, 172, 172*f*
    removing (cats), 26, 26*f*
Collection, blood
    ferret for, 217–218, 218*f*
    rat for, 200, 200*f*
Commanding tone, of voice, 4
Commercial muzzles
    placement of (dogs), 96–98, 96*f*, 98*f*
    removal of (dogs), 98, 98*f*
Commercially prepared muzzles, 96–98
Complications, of restraints, 6
Cover, eye, for horses, 143, 143*f*
Cow
    dairy, 114
    separating from their calf, 110
    sheet bend in, 16
Crook, shepherd's (sheep), 160
Cross tying, of horses, 141, 141*f*

D

Dairy cows, treated in stanchion, 114
Data, physiologic, 231*t*
Defense, pig's primary means of, 178
Defensive "weapons," 3
Dehorning and castration, restraint for
        (goats), 175
Devices
    antikicking (cattle), 126, 126*f*
    movement-limiting (dogs),
        104–105, 104*f*
    restraint (dogs), 96–105
        capture poles, 102, 102*f*
        leather gloves, 102, 102*f*
        muzzles, 96–101
        rope leashes, 102, 102*f*
        towels and blankets, 103, 103*f*
Distraction techniques, for horses, 141–144,
        142–144*f*
    blindfolds as, 143
    caveman pats as, 143
    eye cover as, 143
    hand twitch as, 141
    leg lift as, 144
    rocking an ear as, 141
    skin roll as, 141
Docile, goats, 170
Docking, tail (lambs), 167
Dogs
    aggressive, 57, 62–64, 62*f*, 64*f*
    caged, 58–64, 58*f*
        aggressive dogs, 62–64, 62*f*, 64*f*
        calm dogs, 59–60, 59*f*, 61*f*
        large friendly dogs, 59–60,
            59*f*, 61*f*
        nervous dogs, 62–64, 62*f*, 64*f*
    calm, 59–60, 59*f*, 61*f*
    canine teeth, 56
    and cattle, 110
    gender names, 229
    handling on run, 64–66
        retrieval from run, 64–65, 64*f*
        returning to run, 66, 66*f*

Dogs *(Continued)*
    injured, 57
    large friendly, 59–60, 59*f*, 61*f*
    lifting and carrying, 68–72
        5- to 50-lb, 68–71, 68*f*, 70–71*f*
        more than 50 lbs, 72, 72*f*
    nervous, 57, 62–64, 62*f*, 64*f*
    never have clients restrain them, 56
    no physical reprimand, 56
    old, 57
    physiologic data of, 231*t*
    reprimanding, 56
    restraining large, 83–86, 83*f*
    restraint of, 55–105
        general considerations, 56–57
        general restraint procedures, 73–81
        handling caged dogs, 58–64
        handling dogs in a run, 64–66
        lifting and carrying dogs, 68–72
        movement-limiting devices, 104–105, 104*f*
        potential for injury, 56
        restraining large dogs, 83–86
        restraint devices, 96–105
        restraint for venipuncture, 89–95
        special handling, 56–57
        turning dogs, 88, 88*f*
    turning, 88, 88*f*
Double bow knot, 12, 13*f*
Drawing blood, 93
Duration, in restraint, 6

E

Ear, rocking of, for horses, 141, 142*f*
Ear cleaning, in ferret, 215
Elizabethan collar, in birds, 227
Environment, physical, 5
Equipment
    restraint (cats), 44–52
        blankets, 47, 47*f*
        cat lassos, 52, 52*f*
        cat restraint bags, 48–50, 48*f*, 50*f*
        gauntlets for, 52, 52*f*
        muzzles, 50, 51*f*
        towels, 44–46, 45*f*
    restraint procedures and, 4–5
Examination, restraint for, 170–172, 170*f*
    sheep, 160–164, 161*f*, 163–164*f*
Eye cover, for horses, 143, 143*f*
Eyesight, of horses, 132

F

Feet, lifting, of horses, 151–152, 151–152*f*
Female pigs, 2–3
Ferret, 214–218, 214–216*f*
    blood collection for, 217–218, 218*f*
    gender names, 229
    injections for, 215–217, 216–217*f*
    physiologic data of, 231*t*
    restraint of, 187–218
50-lb dogs, lifting and carrying more than, 72, 72*f*
"Fight or flight" principle, 2
5- to 50-lb dogs, lifting and carrying, 68–71, 68*f*, 70–71*f*
Flanking, of cattle, 128, 129*f*

Flanking a goat, 171, 171*f*
Flight-or-fight response, 5
Foals, restraint of, 156
Fraying, rope in, preventing, 9–10
Friendly dogs, large, 59–60, 59*f*, 61*f*

G

Gauntlets, for cats, 52, 52*f*
Gauze or rope muzzle (dogs), 99–101, 99*f*, 101*f*
Gavages, oral
    for gerbil, 205
    for hamster, 203
    for mouse, 190, 191*f*
    for rat, 196, 196*f*
Gender names, 229
Gerbil, 203–205, 203*f*
    injections for, 205, 205–206*f*
    oral gavage of, 205
    physiologic data of, 231*t*
Gloves
    in capturing, of birds, 223
    heavy (cats), 52
    leather (dogs), 102, 102*f*
Goats
    cannot be treated as sheep, 170
    capture of, 170
    do not tolerate rough treatment, 170
    as docile, 170
    flanking of, 171, 171*f*
    gender names, 229
    physiologic data of, 231*t*
    restraint for examination, 170–172, 170*f*
    restraint of, 169–176
        collars, 172, 172*f*
        for dehorning and castration, 175
        in head, 172, 172*f*
        for hoof trimming, 175, 175*f*
        oral medication, 174, 174*f*
        for venipuncture, 173–174, 173–174*f*
Guinea pig, 207–209, 207*f*
    injections for, 208–209, 208–209*f*
    physiologic data of, 231*t*

H

Half hitch, 8*f*, 20, 20*f*
Halter tie, 14, 15*f*, 140, 140*f*
Halters
    for equine restraint, 136, 137*f*
    rope (cattle), 116–119, 116*f*, 118*f*
    sheep, 160
Hamster, 201–203, 201*f*
    injections for, 203, 203*f*
    oral gavage for, 203
    physiologic data of, 231*t*
Hand twitch, for horses, 141, 142*f*
Handling
    of animals, 3
    special (dogs), 56–57
        aggressive dogs, 57
        injured dogs, 57
        nervous dogs, 57
        old dogs, 57
        pregnant bitches, 57
        puppies, 56–57

Hands, as flexible instruments, 4
"Hanking," 8–9, 9f
Head, restraint of
  cats, 25, 25f
  cattle, 116–120
    nose lead, 120, 121f
    nose ring, 120
    rope halter, 116–119, 116f, 118f
  dogs, 84–86, 84–86f
  goats, 172, 172f
  horses, 141–149
    chain shank for, 149, 149f
    distraction techniques for, 141–144, 142–144f
    twitches for, 145–147, 145–146f, 148f
  swine, 182–184
    hog snare, 182, 183f
Healthy animals, restraint in, 3
Heavy gloves (cats), 52
Herd animals, horses as, 132
Herd instinct, 2
Herding cattle, 108–110, 108f, 110f
Hierarchy, in animals, 3
Hitch
  clove, 21, 21f
  half, 20, 20f
  snubbing, 22, 22f
Hobbles
  for horses, 156
  swine, 184
Hog snare, 182, 183f
Hold, pretzel (cats), 38, 38f
Hondo, lariat with (cattle), 123
Hoof trimming, restraint for (goats), 175, 175f
Hooves, in domestic animals, 3
Horses
  body language of, 132
  calming of, 132
  eyes of, 132
  eyesight of, 132
  gender names, 229
  kicking of, as means of protection, 132
  mouth of, 132
  physiologic data of, 231t
  restraint of, 131–158, 133f
    approaching a horse, 134–138, 135f, 137–138f
    capturing a horse, 134–138, 135f, 137f
    cross tying in, 141, 141f
    foals, 156
    head of, 141–149
    hobbles for, 156
    leading a horse, 139, 139f
    lifting feet in, 151–152, 151–152f
    loading into trailer, 156–158, 156f
    placing a mouth wedge, 153, 153f
    stocks in, 154, 154f
    tail tying in, 155, 155f
    tying a horse, 140, 140f
  sheet bend in, 16
  tail of, 132
  tongue of, 132
Human safety, 2–3
Humane twitch, for horses, 147, 148f
Hurdles (pigs), 178–179, 178f

I
Improper restraint, 2
Inhalation chamber (cats), 52
Injections
  for bird, 225, 225f
  for ferret, 215–217, 216–217f
  for gerbil, 205, 205–206f
  for guinea pig, 208–209, 208–209f
  for hamster, 203, 203f
  for mouse, 192–194, 192f, 194f
  for rabbit, 212, 212f
  for rat, 197–198, 197–198f
  for restrained horses, 133f
Injured dogs, 57
Injury, potential for (dogs), 56
Instincts, pack (dogs), 56
Instructional tone, of voice, 4
Instruments, restraint, 4
Intradermal injections, in guinea pig, 208
Intramuscular injection
  in ferret, 217
  in gerbil, 205
  in guinea pig, 209
  in hamster, 203
  in rabbit, 212
  in rat, 197
Intraperitoneal injection
  in gerbil, 205
  in hamster, 203
  in mouse, 192, 198

J
Jacking, tail (cattle), 126, 127f
Jugular venipuncture
  dogs, 89–90, 89–90f
  restraint for (sheep), 166, 166f

K
Kicking
  cattle, 108
  of horses
    as means of protection, 132
    range, 138
Kid, capture of, 175
Knot tying, 7–22
  equipment maintenance, 8–10, 9–10f
  knots in, types of, 10–22
  terminology of, 8
Knots
  definition of, 8
  types of
    bowline, 16–17, 17f
    bowline on the bight, 18, 18f
    clove hitch, 21, 21f
    half hitch, 20, 20f
    halter tie, 14, 15f
    overhand, 8, 9f
    quick-release knot, 14
    reefer's knot, 12, 12f
    sheet bend, 16, 16f
    snubbing hitch, 22, 22f
    square knot, 10, 11f
    surgeon's knot, 11, 11f
    tomfool knot, 12, 13f
    types of, 10–22

L
Lambs. See also Sheep
  restraint of, 167, 167f
Language, body
  of animals, 4
  of horses, 132
Large animals, 3
Large birds, 222–224, 223f
Large dogs, restraining, 83–86, 83f
Large friendly dogs, 59–60, 59f, 61f
Lariat, with Hondo (cattle), 123
Lassos, cats, 52, 52f
Lateral recumbency
  left (cats), 35, 36f
  placing calf in, 128, 129f
  right (cats), 37, 37f
  two-person, 37, 37f
Lateral restraint
  dogs, 77–79, 77f, 79f
  to standing restraint, 80, 80f
  sternal to (dogs), 81, 82f
Lateral saphenous venipuncture (dogs), 95, 95f
Lead, nose (cattle), 120, 121f
Lead rope, for equine restraint, 135f, 136, 137f
Leading, of horses, 139, 139f
Leashes, rope (dogs), 102, 102f
Leather gloves (dogs), 102, 102f
Left-lateral recumbency (cats), 35, 36f
Leg lift, for horses, 144, 144f
Legs
  lifting (cattle), 123–124, 123–124f
  restraining (cats), 26, 26f
Lifting and carrying dogs, 68–72
  weighing 5 to 50 lbs, 68–71, 68f, 70–71f
  weighing more than 50 lbs, 72, 72f
Lifting feet, of horses, 151–152, 151–152f
Lifting legs (cattle), 123–124, 123–124f
Lifting pigs, carrying or, 180, 181f
Loop, 8, 8f

M
Medical procedures, restraint for, in birds, 224–227
  beak restraint, 227
  cloacal swab, 226, 226f
  Elizabethan collar, 227
  injections, 225, 225f
  oral medications, 224, 224f
  radiography, 227, 227f
  splint application, 226, 226f
  venipuncture, 225, 225f
Medications
  oral
    administration of, in rats, 196
    in birds, 224, 224f
    cattle, 122, 122f
    goats, 174, 174f
    restraint for (sheep), 165, 165f
Mouse, 188–194
  are shy creatures, 188
  cage retrieval and restraint, 188, 189f
  injections for, 192–194, 192f, 194f
  oral gavage, 190, 191f
  physiologic data of, 231t

Mouth, of horses, 132
Mouth wedge, for horses, 153, 153*f*
Movement-limiting devices (dogs),
    104–105, 104*f*
Moving and capturing pigs, 178–179
Muzzles, for cats, 50, 51*f*
Muzzles (dogs)
    commercially prepared, 96–98
        placement of, 96–98, 96*f*, 98*f*
        removal of, 98, 98*f*
    gauze or rope, 99–101, 99*f*, 101*f*

N

Nail trimming, restraining for (cats), 44, 44*f*
Names, gender, 229
Neck chain (goats), 172
Neck strap, for horses, 137*f*
Needle, gavage, for rat, 196
Nervous dogs, 57, 62–64, 62*f*, 64*f*
Nose band, for horses, 137*f*
Nose lead (cattle), 120, 121*f*
Nose ring (cattle), 120
Nylon, or canvas bags (cats), 48

O

Old dogs, 57
Oral gavage
    for gerbil, 205
    for hamster, 203
    for mouse, 190, 191*f*
    for rat, 196, 196*f*
Oral medications
    administration of, in rats, 196
    in birds, 224, 224*f*
    for cattle, 122, 122*f*
    goats, 174, 174*f*
    for restrained horses, 133*f*
Order, pecking, 3
Overhand knot, 8, 9*f*
Owners, no physical reprimands in front of
    (dogs), 56

P

Pack instincts (dogs), 56
Paddles (pigs), 179, 179*f*
Pats, caveman, for horses, 143
Pecking order, 3
Personnel, in restraint, 6
Physical environment, 5
Physiologic data, 231, 231*t*
Pigs. *See also* Swine
    can be vicious animals, 178
    can squeeze through small openings, 178
    carrying or lifting, 180, 181*f*
    female, 2–3
    gender names, 229
    guinea, 207–209, 207*f*
        injections for, 208–209, 208–209*f*
    lifting newborns by tails, 180
    moving and capturing, 178–179
        barriers, 178–179
        bucket and, 179
        hurdles and, 178–179, 178*f*
        paddles and, 179, 179*f*
    primary means of defense, 178
    traits of, 178

Planning, in restraint, 6
Point of balance, in cattle, 108
Poles, capture (dogs), 102, 102*f*
Predator species, 2
Pregnant bitches, 57
Pressure point, in cattle, 108
Pretzel hold (cats), 38, 38*f*
Prey animals (cattle), 108
Principle
    fight or flight, 2
    restraint, 1–6
Procedures
    medical, restraint for, in birds, 224–227
    restraint, 4–5
Protection, kicking as means of, in
    horses, 132
Puppies, 56–57

Q

Quick-release knot, 14, 15*f*

R

Rabbit, 209–213, 210–211*f*
    gender names, 229
    injections for, 212, 212*f*
    physiologic data of, 231*t*
    restraint of, 187–218
    venipuncture of, 213, 213*f*
Radiography, in birds, 227, 227*f*
Rams, battering, 3
Rat, 194–200, 195*f*
    blood collection and, 200, 200*f*
    injections and, 197–198, 197–198*f*
    oral gavages and, 196, 196*f*
    physiologic data of, 231*t*
Recumbency
    left-lateral (cats), 35, 36*f*
    placing calf in lateral, 128, 129*f*
    right-lateral (cats), 37, 37*f*
    two-person (cats), 37, 37*f*
Reefer's knot, 12, 12*f*
Removing a collar (cats), 26, 26*f*
Removing from cage or carrier (cats), 27–29,
    27*f*, 29*f*
Reprimanding dogs, 56
Response, flight-or-fight, 5
Restrain, sheep are easy creatures to, 160
Restraining
    heads, of cats, 25, 25*f*
    legs, of cats, 26, 26*f*
    for nail trimming (cats), 44, 44*f*
Restraining cats
    guidelines for, 25–31
        carrying a cat, 31, 31*f*
        removing a collar, 26, 26*f*
        removing from cage or carrier, 27–30,
            27*f*, 29–30*f*
        restraining heads, 25, 25*f*
        restraining legs, 26, 26*f*
    precautions for, 24–25
Restraining large dogs, 83–86, 83*f*
Restraint bags, cats, 48–50, 48*f*, 50*f*
Restraint devices (dogs), 96–105
    capture poles, 102, 102*f*
    leather gloves, 102, 102*f*

Restraint devices (dogs) *(Continued)*
    muzzles, 96–101
    rope leashes, 102, 102*f*
    towels and blankets, 103, 103*f*
Restraint equipment (cats), 44–52
    blankets, 47, 47*f*
    cat lassos, 52, 52*f*
    cat restraint bags, 48–50, 48*f*, 50*f*
    gauntlets for, 52, 52*f*
    muzzles, 50, 51*f*
    towels, 44–46, 45*f*
Restraint for venipuncture (dogs), 89–95
    cephalic venipuncture, 91, 91*f*
    jugular venipuncture, 89–90, 89–90*f*
    lateral saphenous venipuncture, 95, 95*f*
    tourniquet application, 93, 93*f*
Restraint of cats, 23–53
    applying tourniquets for cephalic
        venipuncture, 41–43, 41–43*f*
    behavior of, 24
    equipment for, 44–52
    guidelines for, 25–31
    for nail trimming, 44, 44*f*
    precautions for restraining cats, 24–25
    restraint for venipunctures, 39, 40*f*
    techniques for, 32–38
Restraint of dogs, 55–105
    general considerations, 56–57
    general restraint procedures, 73–81
    handling caged dogs, 58–64
    handling dogs in a run, 64–66
    lifting and carrying dogs, 68–72
    movement-limiting devices, 104–105, 104*f*
    potential for injury, 56
    restraining large dogs, 83–86
    restraint devices, 96–105
    restraint for venipuncture, 89–95
    special handling, 56–57
    turning dogs, 88, 88*f*
Restraint of ferret, 187–218, 214–216*f*
Restraint of goats, 169–176
    collars, 172, 172*f*
    for dehorning and castration, 175
    for examination, 170–172, 170*f*
    in head, 172, 172*f*
    for hoof trimming, 175, 175*f*
    oral medication, 174, 174*f*
    for venipuncture, 173–174, 173–174*f*
Restraint of head (goats), 172, 172*f*
Restraint of head (swine), 182–184
    hog snare, 182, 183*f*
    snubbing rope, 184
Restraint of rabbits, 187–218, 210–211*f*
Restraint of rodents, 187–218
    gerbil and, 203–205, 203*f*
    guinea pig and, 207–209, 207*f*
    hamster and, 201–203, 201*f*
    mouse and, 188–194
    rat and, 194–200, 195*f*
Restraint of swine, 177–185
    carrying or lifting pigs, 180, 181*f*
    moving and capturing pigs and,
        178–179
    restraint of head, 182–184
    whole-body restraint, 184

Restraint procedures, general (dogs), 73–81
  lateral restraint, 77–79, 77f, 79f
  lateral restraint to standing restraint, 80, 80f
  standing restraint, 73–74, 73–74f
  sternal restraint, 75–77, 75–77f
  sternal to lateral restraint, 81, 82f
Restraint techniques (cats), 32–38
  cat's left side will touch table, 35, 36f
  cat's right side will touch table, 37, 37f
  left-lateral recumbency, 35, 36f
  pretzel hold, 38, 38f
  standing restraints, 32, 32f
  sternal restraint, 33, 33–34f
  two-person lateral recumbency, 37, 37f
Restraints
  on animals, 2
  beak, 227
  of birds, 219–227
    capturing, 220–224
    for medical procedures, 224–227
    transport to clinic, 220
  cage retrieval and (mice), 188, 189f
  of calves, 128
    flanking of, 128, 129f
  for castration (lambs), 167
  of cattle, 107–130
    antikicking devices for, 126, 126f
    of calves, 128
    in chutes and stanchions, 111–114, 111f, 114f
    of heads, 116–120
    herding of, 108–110, 108f, 110f
    lifting legs in, 123–124, 123–124f
    oral medications for, 122, 122f
    using tails, 126–127
  chemical, 3, 5
  chemical (cats), 52
  in chutes and stanchions (cattle), 111–114, 111f, 114f
  circumstances for, 5–6
  complications of, 6
  considerations for, 2–5
  definition of, 2
  for dehorning and castration (goats), 175
  equipment, 4–5
  for examination (goats), 170–172, 170f
  for examination (sheep), 160–164, 161f, 163–164f
  of head (horses), 141–149
    chain shank for, 149, 149f
    distraction techniques for, 141–144, 142–144f
    twitches for, 145–147, 145–146f, 148f
  of head (cattle), 116–120
    nose lead, 120, 121f
    nose ring, 120
    rope halter, 116–119, 116f, 118f
  of head (dogs), 84–86, 84–86f
  for hoof trimming (goats), 175, 175f
  of horses, 131–158, 133f
    approaching a horse, 134–138, 135f, 137–138f
    capturing a horse, 134–138, 135f, 137f
    cross tying in, 141, 141f
    foals, 156

Restraints (Continued)
  head of, 141–149
  hobbles for, 156
  leading a horse, 139, 139f
  lifting feet in, 151–152, 151–152f
  loading into trailer, 156–158, 156f
  placing a mouth wedge, 153, 153f
  stocks in, 154, 154f
  tail tying in, 155, 155f
  tying a horse, 140, 140f
  improper, 2
  instruments, 4
  for jugular venipuncture (sheep), 166, 166f
  of lambs, 167, 167f
  lateral (dogs), 77–81, 77f, 79–80f, 82f
  for medications, 165, 165f
  mildest form of, 2
  moderate form of, 2
  principles of, 1–6
  procedures, 4–5
  restrictive form of, 2
  of sheep, 159–168
    capturing of, 160, 160f
    for examination, 160–164, 161f, 163–164f
    for jugular venipuncture, 166, 166f
    of lambs, 167, 167f
    for medications, 165, 165f
  standing (cats), 32, 32f
  standing (dogs), 73–74, 73–74f, 80, 80f
  sternal (cats), 33, 33–34f
  sternal (dogs), 75–77, 75–77f
  for tail docking (lambs), 167
  techniques, learning, 2
  using tails (cattle), 126–127
    tail jacking, 126, 127f
    tail tying, 127, 128f
  for venipuncture (cats), 39, 40f
  for venipuncture (goats), 173–174, 173–174f
Retrieval and restraint, cage (mouse), 188, 189f
Retrieval from run (dogs), 64–65, 64f
Returning to cages or carrier (cats), 30, 30f
Returning to run (dogs), 66, 66f
Right-lateral recumbency (cats), 37, 37f
Ring, nose (cattle), 120
Rocking, an ear, for horses, 141, 142f
Rodents, restraint of, 187–218
  gerbil and, 203–205, 203f
  guinea pig and, 207–209, 207f
  hamster and, 201–203, 201f
  mouse and, 188–194
  rat and, 194–200, 195f
Roll, skin, for horses, 141, 142f
Rope. See also Knot tying
  for equine restraint, 135f, 136, 137f
  snubbing (swine), 184
Rope halter (cattle), 116–119, 116f, 118f
Rope leashes (dogs), 102, 102f
Rope muzzle, gauze or (dogs), 99–101, 99f, 101f
Rope twitch, for horses, 147
Rough treatment, goats not tolerating, 170

Run
  handling dogs on, 64–66
  retrieval from (dogs), 64–65, 64f
  returning to (dogs), 66, 66f

S
Safety
  animal, 3–4
  considerations, 2–4
  human, 2–3
Saphenous venipuncture, lateral (dogs), 95, 95f
Setting, in restraint, 5
Shank, chain, for horses, 149, 149f
Sheep
  always work with assurance around, 160
  are easy creatures to restrain, 160
  capturing of, 160, 160f
  with full coat of wool, 160
  gender names, 229
  goats cannot be treated like, 170
  physiologic data of, 231t
  restraint of, 159–168
    capturing of, 160, 160f
    for examination, 160–164, 161f, 163–164f
    for jugular venipuncture, 166, 166f
    of lambs, 167, 167f
    for medications, 165, 165f
Sheet bend, 16, 16f
Shepherd's crook (sheep), 160
Shy creatures, mice are, 188
Single bow knot, 12, 12f
Skin roll, for horses, 141, 142f
Small birds, 220–222, 221–222f
Snare, hog, 182, 183f
Snubbing hitch, 22, 22f
Snubbing ropes (swine), 184
Soothing tone, of voice, 4
Sows (female pigs), 2–3
Special handling (dogs), 56–57
  aggressive dogs, 57
  injured dogs, 57
  nervous dogs, 57
  old dogs, 57
  pregnant bitches, 57
  puppies, 56–57
Splint application, in birds, 226, 226f
Square knot, 10, 11f
Stallions, 3
Stanchions
  dairy cows treated in, 114
  restraint in chutes and (cattle), 111–114, 111f, 114f
Standing part, of rope, 8
Standing restraint
  cats, 32, 32f
  dogs, 73–74, 73–74f
  lateral restraint to (dogs), 80, 80f
Sternal restraint
  cats, 33, 33–34f
  dogs, 75–77, 75–77f
Sternal to lateral restraint (dogs), 81, 82f
Stocks, for horses, 154, 154f
Storing ropes, 8–9

Stress
   in birds, 220
   in healthy animals, 3
Stud shank, for horses, 149
Subcutaneous injections
   in ferret, 215
   in gerbil, 205
   in mouse, 192, 203
Surgeon's knot, 11, 11*f*
Swab, cloacal, in birds, 226, 226*f*
Swine
   physiologic data of, 231*t*
   restraint of, 177–185
      carrying or lifting pigs, 180, 181*f*
      moving and capturing pigs and,
         178–179
      restraint of head, 182–184

T

Table
   cat's left side will touch, 35, 36*f*
   cat's right side will touch, 37, 37*f*
Tail docking, restraint for (lambs), 167
Tail jacking (cattle), 126, 127*f*
Tail tie, 16
Tail tying
   of cattle, 127, 128*f*
   for horses, 155, 155*f*
Tails
   indicating a horse's attitude, 132
   lifting newborns by, 180
   likely amputated (sheep), 164
   restraint using (cattle), 126–127
      tail jacking, 126, 127*f*
      tail tying, 127, 128*f*
Techniques, for distraction, of horses,
      141–144, 142–144*f*
   blindfolds as, 143
   caveman pats as, 143
   eye cover as, 143
   hand twitch as, 141
   leg lift as, 144

Techniques, for distraction, of horses
      (Continued)
   rocking an ear as, 141
   skin roll as, 141
Techniques, restraint (cats), 32–38, 33–34*f*
   cat's left side will touch table, 35
   cat's right side will touch table, 37, 37*f*
   left-lateral recumbency, 35, 36*f*
   pretzel hold, 38, 38*f*
   right-lateral recumbency, 37, 37*f*
   standing restraints, 32, 32*f*
   two-person lateral recumbency, 37, 37*f*
Teeth, in domestic animals, 3
Temperature, 5
   in restraint, 5
   taking of, in restrained horses, 133*f*
Terminology, of knot tying, 8, 8–10*f*
Throw, 8, 9*f*
Tie
   halter, 14, 15*f*
   tail, 16
Time, in restraint, 5
Tomfool knot, 12, 13*f*
Tongue, of horses, 132
Tourniquets
   application (dogs), 93, 93*f*
   applying for cephalic venipuncture (cats),
      41–43, 41–43*f*
Towels, 103, 103*f*
   cats, 44–46, 45*f*
Trailer, loading into, of horses, 156–158, 156*f*
Traits of pigs, 178
Transport to clinic, in restraint of birds, 220
Treatment, goats do not tolerate rough, 170
Trimming
   restraining for nails (cats), 44, 44*f*
   restraint for hoof (goats), 175, 175*f*
Trough (swine), 184, 185*f*
Turning dogs, 88, 88*f*
Twitches
   hand, for horses, 141, 142*f*
   for horses, 145–147, 145–146*f*, 148*f*

Two-person lateral recumbency
      (cats), 37, 37*f*
Tying
   cross, of horses, 141, 141*f*
   of horses, 140, 140*f*
   knot, 7–22
   tail (cattle), 127, 128*f*
   tail (horses), 155, 155*f*

U

Unraveling, rope in, preventing, 9–10
Unrestrained large animals, 3
   crushed by, 3

V

Veins, cephalic (goats), 173
Venipuncture
   applying tourniquets for cephalic (cats),
      41–43, 41–43*f*
   in birds, 225, 225*f*
   cephalic (dogs), 91, 91*f*
   jugular (dogs), 89–90, 89–90*f*
   lateral saphenous (dogs), 95, 95*f*
   of rabbit, 213, 213*f*
   restraint for jugular (sheep), 166, 166*f*
   restraints for (cats), 39, 40*f*
   restraints for (dogs), 89–95
      cephalic venipuncture, 91, 91*f*
      jugular venipuncture, 89–90, 89–90*f*
      lateral saphenous venipuncture, 95, 95*f*
      tourniquet application, 93, 93*f*
   restraints for (goats), 173–174, 173–174*f*
Vicious animals, pigs can be, 178
Voice, 4–5

W

Weapons, defensive, 3
Wedge, mouth, for horses, 153, 153*f*
Whole-body, restraint, 184
   hobbles, 184
   trough, 184, 185*f*
Wool, sheep with full coat of, 160